REMARKABLE BLACK BABY NAMES

First published in Great Britain in 2022 by Penny's House Publishing.

A CIP catalogue record for this title is available from the British Library

Paperback ISBN 9781739880705
Ebook ISBN 9781739880712

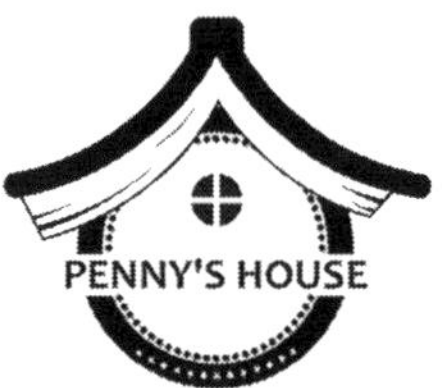

pennyshousepublishing.com

REMARKABLE BLACK BABY NAMES

The Perfect Baby Name Book
To Find Powerful & Inspired
Names With Their Meanings

TONY & SHARLENE CHANCE

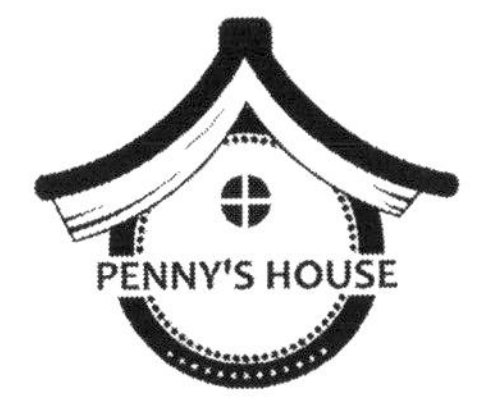

DEDICATION

This book is dedicated to our firstborn son Omari. May you forever flourish ♥

CONTENTS

INTRODUCTION

Congratulations - you're having a baby!

Whilst we were writing this book, it occurred to us that it doesn't matter where you're from or what you do, we all have to go through the process of deciding on a name for our baby. And, for most of us, it's a pretty tough task. "I get one shot at this...can't mess it up" - the harsh reality!

When we were choosing our son's name, it took the whole pregnancy plus another 2 months (our son was born during the pandemic so we (LUCKILY) had longer to register him than normal). The challenge - to find a name that sounded nice, that couldn't be abbreviated to something ridiculous or offensive and most importantly, that was meaningful and reflected our hopes for his life. Trawling the internet and searching through outdated websites for name inspo is hard and frankly, not that inspiring. Finally though, we agreed on Omari. And he's such an Omari - flourishing!

HOWEVER, if I had been given this book at that time, there would have been so many more GOOD options. I think he might have even ended up with a Zyan!

Point is, we made this book to be an easier, more inspiring solution to finding a name for your baby that feels...right! A powerful, inspired, remarkable name fitting for the beautiful baby you're about to welcome into this world.

We've carefully selected thousands of names and categorized them into 11 simple categories so you can focus on what matters most to YOU.

Unlike other baby name books, this book is Black first! We built an amazing team of Black parents from all over the world to curate over 3000 names that have cultural significance or appeal within the Black community. Obviously, we're not saying all 3000+ will appeal to everyone in the community but you were first in mind when all of the names were curated.

We also included the meanings of every name in this book. Knowing the meaning of a name makes it so much more meaningful to you and one day, to your child as well. Also, it's actually really interesting to read through name meanings. We didn't include pronunciations because - who gets to decide how to say something right? That's YOUR choice. Besides if you're in America, you'll more than likely pronounce half these names differently to if you're in the UK. There's no wrong or right on that front.

Don't forget to use the notes section (at the back of this book) to jot down the name and page numbers you like. That shortlist gonna be looking real good, real soon! You‘ve got this.

Whatever name you choose, may you and your baby be happy and healthy always x

HOW TO USE THIS BOOK

First things first. This is not a book that you HAVE to read end to end. We were very careful to design a book that allows you to go where your heart (or head) leads and take it from there.

This book is split into 3 main sections:

1. Names for Girls
2. Names for Boy
3. Gender-Neutral Names

Each section is then split into 11 different categories:

1. Positive Meaning
2. Space & Nature
3. African Origin
4. Biblical
5. Influential People
6. Popular
7. Arabic
8. African American
9. Modern
10. Classic
11. Religious

Each category is listed in alphabetical order. Each name includes the meaning and origin (if known). If you're looking in the Influential People category, it'll also show some details about the influential person the name refers to.

The simplest way to use this book is to start in the relevant section then browse the categories that you connect with most. When you find a name that gives you good vibes, use the Notes section to jot it down with its page number.

Some tips, thoughts and considerations when choosing your perfect baby names:

The "Say It Out LOUD" Test:

When we were choosing our son's name - we used to call it out! Not only is that great practice for something you'll inevitably end up doing ALL day but it also helps you see how it fits in real life. Does it feel comfortable? Does it sound "right"?

How Will People Abbreviate It & What Nicknames Will They Give?

Names always end up getting abbreviated. I (Sharlene) really liked the name Orion but Tony rejected it because he thought people would just end up calling the baby "Ryan". Lol. If a likely abbreviation really bothers you, the name might not be ideal.

Nicknames are also something you may think about when choosing a name. Our son's name is Omari Junior so we knew he may end up with the nickname "OJ" (Orange Juice). We could live with that but some names offered up nicknames we couldn't bear the idea of our son living with!

Our tip: spend a short amount of time doing a little brainstorm of nicknames and abbreviations you might associate with your shortlisted names. Don't overthink it though!

Alternative Spellings & Pronunciations

I've spent my life saying "Sharlene - spelt with an S". I'm someone with an alternative spelling and although my name is constantly spelt wrong, I love the fact that it's spelt differently.

We've typically only included one spelling in this book and we stayed away from telling you how to pronounce a name. We think these are personal decisions and one where there is no wrong or right. The challenges of non-standard spelling or pronunciation are definitely something worth factoring in (we definitely wrote some names down and asked friends how they would pronounce it to make sure the result was nothing crazy) but it is a personal decision and an element you can play around with to add some individuality and uniqueness if that's what you're looking for.

Double Meanings

Many names have more than one meaning. To reduce the stress and overwhelm that this can cause, we only included one meaning in most cases (usually the most common).

Which Gender?

Names have been categorized under the gender which most commonly applies. This doesn't mean it couldn't be used for the opposite gender - this is a personal decision. There is also a section of Gender Neutral names but again this isn't exclusive and any name featured in any section could be considered gender-neutral.

Why You'll See Some Names Once Than Once

As you browse this book, you'll see the same names feature more than once. We have put names in ALL the categories they apply. This is just so you don't miss out on anything if you decide not to check through every single category.

Some pointers - if you want them:

These are some of the things that helped us to make a choice:

1. Start in a category that reflects your interests/passions/beliefs
2. Choose 2-4 first initials you like best (start with those letters in the category you're browsing)
3. Be open-minded and enjoy the process!

If your baby's name is a joint decision, a really helpful way to get to an agreement was to start by agreeing on the categories and first initials. This doesn't lead to a guaranteed agreement but it will narrow the gap and hopefully make your shortlists more aligned!

GIRLS' NAMES A-Z BY CATEGORY

POSITIVE MEANING

"Happiness is a mood. Positivity is a mindset."

Girl ♀

A

Abigail
Meaning: Cause of joy
Origin: Hebrew

Abiola
Meaning: Born in honor/wealth
Origin: African–Nigeria

Adelaide
Meaning: Noble person
Origin: German

Adeline
Meaning: Noble
Origin: French

Adira
Meaning: Strong, powerful
Origin: Hebrew

Adora
Meaning: Beloved, adored
Origin: French

Afyia
Meaning: Good health
Origin: Arabic

Akeila
Meaning: Brilliant, intelligent, gifted
Origin: Russian

Akilah
Meaning: Intelligent
Origin: Arabic

Akira
Meaning: Bright, intelligent, clear
Origin: Japanese

Alaina
Meaning: Precious
Origin: Hawaiian

Alamea
Meaning: Precious
Origin: Hawaiian

Alexa
Meaning: Defender of mankind
Origin: Greek

Alexandria
Meaning: Defender of mankind
Origin: Greek

Aliyah
Meaning: Ascending, exalted, elevated
Origin: Arabic

Allyson
Meaning: Noble
Origin: German

Althea
Meaning: Healer
Origin: Greek

Amalhe
Meaning: The beautiful one
Origin: African

Amandla
Meaning: Power
Origin: African–South Africa

Amara
Meaning: Loveable
Origin: Latin

Amarika
Meaning: Everlasting
Origin: Sanskrit

Ambrose
Meaning: Immortal
Origin: Latin

Amena
Meaning: Honest
Origin: Arabic

Amina
Meaning: Honest, faithful
Origin: Arabic

Amy
Meaning: Beloved
Origin: French

Angela
Meaning: Heavenly messenger
Origin: Greek

Aniyah
Meaning: God favors
Origin: Hebrew

Annika
Meaning: Grace
Origin: Hebrew

Asha
Meaning: Hope
Origin: African–Swahili

Asher
Meaning: Happy, blessed
Origin: Hebrew

Augusta
Meaning: Great, magnificent
Origin: Latin

Austin
Meaning: Great
Origin: Unknown

Ayira
Meaning: The chosen one
Origin: African

B

Bali
Meaning: Strength
Origin: Indonesian

Bari'ah
Meaning: Excelling
Origin: Arabic

Beatrice
Meaning: She who makes happy
Origin: Unknown

Beau
Meaning: Beautiful
Origin: French

Bella
Meaning: Beautiful
Origin: Latin

Benedicta
Meaning: Blessed
Origin: Latin

Bennett
Meaning: The blessed one
Origin: English

Bernadette
Meaning: Brave as a bear
Origin: French

Bernadine
Meaning: Brave as a bear
Origin: French

Bernice
Meaning: Victory, conquest, success, mastery
Origin: Greek

Beyoncé
Meaning: Beyond others
Origin: Creole

Bisa
Meaning: Greatly loved
Origin: African

Bobby/Bobbie
Meaning: Famous, bright
Origin: German

Breana, Brianna
Meaning: Noble, high
Origin: Irish

Bree
Meaning: Noble, power
Origin: Irish

Bridgitte
Meaning: Exalted one
Origin: Unknown

C

Cairo
Meaning: Victorious
Origin: Arabic

Calixta
Meaning: Most beautiful
Origin: Greek

Calla
Meaning: Beautiful
Origin: Greek

Cari
Meaning: Beloved
Origin: Welsh

Carissa
Meaning: Beloved, grace
Origin: Greek

Cassandra
Meaning: Shining, excelling
Origin: Greek

Celeste
Meaning: Heavenly
Origin: Latin

Chalondra
Meaning: Smart
Origin: African

Chara
Meaning: Joy, happiness
Origin: Greek

Cherise
Meaning: Precious one
Origin: French

Cheryl
Meaning: Beloved
Origin: French

Clara
Meaning: Brilliant, bright
Origin: Latin

Cleona
Meaning: Father's glory
Origin: Greek

Coco
Meaning: Celebrated one
Origin: Greek

Comfort
Meaning: To strengthen greatly
Origin: Unknown

D

Damita
Meaning: Little noble woman
Origin: Spanish

Davina
Meaning: Beloved
Origin: Scottish

Dayo
Meaning: Happiness has come
Origin: African

De-Andra
Meaning: Defender of mankind, divine
Origin: African American

Desirae
Meaning: Much desired
Origin: French

Devisha
Meaning: Peace, intelligent
Origin: Indian

Diane
Meaning: Divine
Origin: Latin

Dina
Meaning: Fair, judged
Origin: Hebrew

Dintle
Meaning: Beauty
Origin: African

Dionne
Meaning: Divine
Origin: Greek

Dova
Meaning: Peace
Origin: Hebrew

Duchess
Meaning: Leader
Origin: Latin

E

Eartha
Meaning: Worldly/Earth
Origin: English

Effie
Meaning: Well-spoken
Origin: Greek

Elayah
Meaning: Gifted with prosperity
Origin: African American

Electra
Meaning: Shining
Origin: Greek

Ellen
Meaning: Shining Light
Origin: Greek

Elu
Meaning: Beautiful
Origin: Native American

Emelia
Meaning: Industrious
Origin: Latin

Emerson
Meaning: Brave, powerful
Origin: British

Evangelia
Meaning: Bringer of good news
Origin: Greek

Evelyn
Meaning: Desired
Origin: English

F

Fana
Meaning: One who provides light
Origin: African

Faustina
Meaning: Fortunate
Origin: Unknown

Fidelia
Meaning: Faithful
Origin: Latin

Frida
Meaning: Peace
Origin: German

G

Galena
Meaning: Calm
Origin: Greek

Gene
Meaning: Born lucky
Origin: Greek

Ghadah
Meaning: Beautiful
Origin: Arabic

Gillian
Meaning: Youthful
Origin: Unknown

Gimbya
Meaning: Princess
Origin: African

Gloria
Meaning: Glory
Origin: Latin

Grace
Meaning: Charm, goodness, generosity
Origin: Latin

Gracilyn
Meaning: Grace
Origin: Latin

Gwen
Meaning: Fair
Origin: Welsh

Gwendolyn
Meaning: Blessed
Origin: Welsh

Gwenith/Gwyneth
Meaning: Happy
Origin: Welsh

Gzifa
Meaning: Peaceful one
Origin: African

H

Habibah
Meaning: Beloved
Origin: Arabic

Halima
Meaning: Patient
Origin: Arabic

Harriet
Meaning: Home Ruler
Origin: English

Hera
Meaning: Protectress
Origin: Greek

Hope
Meaning: Expectation
Origin: English

I

Ida
Meaning: Industrious one
Origin: German

Ifama
Meaning: All is well
Origin: African

Ifeoma
Meaning: A good thing
Origin: African

Ifiok
Meaning: Wisdom
Origin: African

Ingrid
Meaning: Beautiful
Origin: Scandinavian

Irene
Meaning: Peace
Origin: Unknown

Isis
Meaning: Throne
Origin: Egyptian

Ivy
Meaning: Faithfulness
Origin: English

J

Jaha
Meaning: Dignified
Origin: Swahili

Jahzara
Meaning: Blessed princess
Origin: African

Jala
Meaning: Shining, bringing to light
Origin: Arabic

Jaya
Meaning: Victorious
Origin: Indian

Jazz
Meaning: Derived from Jasmine meaning gift from God
Origin: Persian

Jovita
Meaning: Happy
Origin: Latin

Joya
Meaning: Joy
Origin: Latin

Juliet
Meaning: Youthful
Origin: French/English

K

Kalei
Meaning: The beloved
Origin: Hawaiian

Kalisha
Meaning: Fortunate woman
Origin: Latin

Kamea
Meaning: The one and only
Origin: Hawaiian

Kanza
Meaning: Treasure
Origin: Arabic

Karah
Meaning: Beloved
Origin: Latin

Karasi
Meaning: Full of life and wisdom
Origin: African

Karine
Meaning: Pure
Origin: Unknown

Karlene
Meaning: Womanly strength
Origin: German

Kasi
Meaning: Shining
Origin: Indian

Kate
Meaning: Pure
Origin: Greek

Katlego
Meaning: Success
Origin: African

Katleho
Meaning: Success
Origin: African

Kay
Meaning: Pure
Origin: Unknown

Kelis
Meaning: Beautiful
Origin: American

Kendria
Meaning: Greatest champion
Origin: Welsh

Keshon
Meaning: God is merciful
Origin: English

Kiana
Meaning: Divine
Origin: Hawaiian

Kianga
Meaning: Sunshine
Origin: African

Kimani
Meaning: Adventurer
Origin: African

Kinta
Meaning: Laughter
Origin: Aboriginal

Kioko
Meaning: Born with happiness
Origin: Japanese

Kira
Meaning: Ruler
Origin: Greek

Kirabo
Meaning: Gift from God
Origin: African

Kisembo
Meaning: Gift
Origin: African–Uganda

Kya
Meaning: Diamond in the sky
Origin: African

Kylie
Meaning: Graceful, beautiful
Origin: Gaelic

L

La-Verne
Meaning: Alder tree grove
Origin: French

Lacrecia/Lacricia
Meaning: Succeed
Origin: Latin

Lamia
Meaning: Radiant
Origin: Arabic

Laquisha
Meaning: Joyful, happy
Origin: English

Larissa
Meaning: Cheerful
Origin: Greek

Lateisha
Meaning: Joyful, happy
Origin: English

Latifah
Meaning: Kind, gentle
Origin: Arabic

Latoria
Meaning: Victorious one
Origin: Spanish

Latoyah
Meaning: Victory
Origin: Unknown

Latreece
Meaning: Noble
Origin: American

Latricia
Meaning: Noble
Origin: American/Latin

Lerato
Meaning: Song of my soul, to adore a person
Origin: African

Lesia
Meaning: Noble
Origin: Latin

Lewa
Meaning: Beautiful
Origin: African

Lois
Meaning: Most desirable
Origin: Greek

Lucinda
Meaning: Light
Origin: Latin

Lucy
Meaning: Light
Origin: Latin

Lux
Meaning: Light
Origin: Latin

M

Mable
Meaning: Lovable, loving
Origin: French

Madea
Meaning: Matriarch of the family
Origin: African

Magic
Meaning: Full of wonder
Origin: American

Maha
Meaning: Beautiful eyes
Origin: Arabic

Mahari
Meaning: Forgiver
Origin: African

Maia
Meaning: Great
Origin: Latin

Maisha
Meaning: Alive and well
Origin: Arabic

Makena
Meaning: Happy one
Origin: African

Malaika
Meaning: Angel
Origin: African

Malaya
Meaning: Free
Origin: Filipino

Malene
Meaning: Magnificent
Origin: German

Maletsasi
Meaning: Sunshine
Origin: African

Malia
Meaning: Peaceful, calm
Origin: Hawaiian

Malika
Meaning: Queen
Origin: Arabic

Mamello
Meaning: Patience
Origin: African

Mandisa
Meaning: Sweet
Origin: African

Maram
Meaning: Desire, wish
Origin: Arabic

Mariama
Meaning: Gift of God
Origin: African–West African

Marihah
Meaning: Exceedingly happy, joyful, cheerful
Origin: Arabic

Martina
Meaning: Warrior
Origin: Latin

Melcia
Meaning: Ambitious
Origin: Teutonic

Melitte
Meaning: Full of grace
Origin: African–Tigrinya of Eritrea and Ethiopia

Mhina
Meaning: Delightful
Origin: African–Bakongo of Zaire

Mila
Meaning: Favored
Origin: Spanish

Mina
Meaning: Love
Origin: German

Minerva
Meaning: Intellect
Origin: Latin

Monifa
Meaning: Lucky
Origin: African–Egyptian

Monisha
Meaning: Intellectual
Origin: Indian

Mugisa / Mugisha
Meaning: Blessing
Origin: African

Mukai
Meaning: Most beautiful
Origin: Arabic

Mya
Meaning: Beloved, great
Origin: Greek

N

Naa
Meaning: Queen
Origin: African

Nabulungi
Meaning: Beautiful
Origin: African

Nacala
Meaning: Peace, Tranquility
Origin: African–Lomwe of Mozambique

Nadia
Meaning: Hope
Origin: Slavic

Nadine
Meaning: Hope
Origin: French

Naeemah
Meaning: Happiness, comfort
Origin: Arabic

Nailah
Meaning: Successful
Origin: Arabic

Nala
Meaning: Successful
Origin: African

Naomi
Meaning: Pleasantness
Origin: Hebrew

Nayo
Meaning: Joyful
Origin: African–Yoruba

Neo/Neyo
Meaning: Gift
Origin: African Origin/American

Niesha
Meaning: Likely derived from Aisha meaning full of life
Origin: Arabic

Nikeisha
Meaning: Likely derived from Keisha meaning great joy
Origin: American

Nikita
Meaning: Unconquered, victory
Origin: Greek

Nikki
Meaning: Victory of the people
Origin: American

Nora
Meaning: Honor, light
Origin: Greek/Latin

Nsombi
Meaning: Abundant joy
Origin: African–Central region

Ntsako
Meaning: Joy, happiness
Origin: African–Tsonga of Central Africa

Ntsumi
Meaning: Angel
Origin: African–Xitsonga

Nyakio
Meaning: Hard Working
Origin: African–Kikuyu of Kenya

Nyesha
Meaning: Pure
Origin: American

Nyla
Meaning: Champion
Origin: British

O

Obioma
Meaning: Kind hearted
Origin: African–Nigeria

Omorose
Meaning: Beautiful
Origin: African

Onika
Meaning: A courageous soldier
Origin: Sanskrit

Orlando
Meaning: Famous throughout the land
Origin: Unknown

Oseye
Meaning: One who is happy
Origin: African

P

Pamela
Meaning: All honey, sweetness
Origin: English/Greek

Pandora
Meaning: All gifts, talented
Origin: Greek

Panya
Meaning: Crowned with laurels
Origin: Latin

Phenyo
Meaning: Victory
Origin: African–Botswana

Phylicia
Meaning: Lucky, fortunate
Origin: Latin

Precious
Meaning: Of great worth, expensive
Origin: Latin

Q

Qadira
Meaning: Powerful, able
Origin: Arabic

Qianna
Meaning: Gracious
Origin: English

Quinlan
Meaning: Very strong
Origin: Irish

Quisha
Meaning: Having a beautiful mind
Origin: American

Quisilla
Meaning: Lovely, pretty
Origin: Indian

R

Raina
Meaning: Queen
Origin: Latin/Slavic

Reagan
Meaning: Little king
Origin: Irish

Reese
Meaning: Enthusiastic
Origin: Welsh

Regina
Meaning: Queen
Origin: Latin

Reilly
Meaning: Courageous
Origin: Irish

Reina
Meaning: Queen
Origin: Latin

Renee
Meaning: Reborn
Origin: French

Rihanna
Meaning: Great queen
Origin: Irish

Ronice
Meaning: Joy is mine
Origin: Hebrew

Ronna
Meaning: Bringing victory
Origin: American

Roshawna
Meaning: Shining light
Origin: Sanskrit

Rowena
Meaning: Fame and happiness
Origin: German

Royal
Meaning: The king
Origin: English

Rufaro
Meaning: Happiness
Origin: Africa–Zimbabwe

Rumi
Meaning: Beauty
Origin: Japanese

Russom
Meaning: One who is a leader
Origin: Swahili

Ruvarashe
Meaning: God's flower
Origin: Africa–Zimbabwe

S

Sada
Meaning: Pure one
Origin: Japanese

Sadie
Meaning: Princess
Origin: Hebrew

Safiya/Saffiyyah
Meaning: Pure
Origin: Arabic

Saidah
Meaning: Fortunate
Origin: Arabic

Saira
Meaning: Princess
Origin: Hebrew

Salama
Meaning: Peace
Origin: Arabic

Salma
Meaning: Peaceful
Origin: Arabic

Samantha
Meaning: Listener
Origin: English

Samora
Meaning: Guarded by God
Origin: Hebrew

Sanya
Meaning: Brilliant
Origin: Arabic

Sanyu
Meaning: Happiness
Origin: African

Saphir
Meaning: Sapphire, gem
Origin: Biblical

Sara
Meaning: Princess
Origin: Hebrew

Sarah
Meaning: Noblewoman, Princess
Origin: Hebrew

Sarai
Meaning: My lady, princess
Origin: Hebrew

Saran
Meaning: Joy
Origin: African

Sarudzai
Meaning: The chosen one
Origin: African

Sekai
Meaning: One who brings laughter and great joy
Origin: African

Selam
Meaning: Peace
Origin: African

Selma
Meaning: Peaceful
Origin: Arabic

Semira
Meaning: From Heaven
Origin: Hebrew

Serena
Meaning: Tranquil
Origin: Latin

Serenity
Meaning: Peaceful
Origin: Latin

Serwa
Meaning: Noblewoman
Origin: African

Shakia
Meaning: Good-looking
Origin: Arabic

Shakila
Meaning: Beautiful
Origin: Arabic

Shalesia
Meaning: Lively
Origin: Unknown

Shalonna
Meaning: Lioness
Origin: Unknown

Shamica/Shamika
Meaning: Majestic
Origin: American

Shanae
Meaning: God is gracious
Origin: Hebrew

Shandra
Meaning: She who outshines the stars
Origin: Indian

Shaneta
Meaning: Gracious
Origin: American

Shania
Meaning: Beautiful
Origin: Unknown

Shanice
Meaning: God is merciful
Origin: Hebrew

Shaniqua
Meaning: Gift of God
Origin: African American

Shanique
Meaning: God is gracious
Origin: American

Shaqueela
Meaning: Beautiful
Origin: Arabic

Sharifa
Meaning: Noble
Origin: Arabic

Shauna
Meaning: God is gracious
Origin: Irish

Shereen
Meaning: Sweet, pleasant
Origin: Arabic

Shiphrah
Meaning: Beautiful
Origin: Hebrew

Shireen
Meaning: Sweet
Origin: Persian

Shukura
Meaning: Grateful
Origin: Egyptian

Sian
Meaning: God's precious gift
Origin: Welsh

Sima
Meaning: Treasure
Origin: Hebrew

Skylar
Meaning: Scholar
Origin: Dutch

Sonia
Meaning: Wisdom
Origin: Greek

Soraya
Meaning: Gem, jewel
Origin: Persian

Ssanyu
Meaning: Joy
Origin: African

Subria
Meaning: Patience
Origin: African

Sula
Meaning: Peace
Origin: Hebrew

Syandene
Meaning: Punctual
Origin: African

T

Tabia
Meaning: Talented
Origin: African

Taheisha
Meaning: Joy
Origin: American

Taisha
Meaning: Alive and well
Origin: Sanskrit

Takeisha
Meaning: Derived from Keisha meaning great joy
Origin: American

Takiyah
Meaning: Righteous
Origin: American

Takunda
Meaning: We have overcome
Origin: African

Talayah
Meaning: Golden ray of sun
Origin: Arabic

Taleisha
Meaning: Blooming life
Origin: African American

Talisa
Meaning: Of noble birth
Origin: Spanish

Tameca
Meaning: Sweet
Origin: American

Tamecia
Meaning: Sweet
Origin: American

Tanasha
Meaning: Reigning queen
Origin: African

Tangela
Meaning: Angel
Origin: Greek

Tapanga
Meaning: Sweet
Origin: African

Taraji
Meaning: Hope
Origin: African

Tariro
Meaning: Hope
Origin: African

Tata
Meaning: Cheerful
Origin: Unknown

Tatiana
Meaning: Fairy princess
Origin: Latin

Tazara
Meaning: One who is elegant
Origin: Arabic

Tene
Meaning: One who is much loved
Origin: African

Teona
Meaning: Princess
Origin: Jamaican

Terehasa
Meaning: Blessed
Origin: African

Teshi
Meaning: Cheerful
Origin: African

Thalia
Meaning: Flourishing
Origin: Greek

Thandiwe
Meaning: Beloved
Origin: African

Thea
Meaning: Goddess
Origin: Greek

Thema
Meaning: Queen
Origin: African

Tiffany
Meaning: Manifestation of God
Origin: Greek

Titilayo
Meaning: Eternal happiness
Origin: African

Tiwa
Meaning: One who owns the crown
Origin: African

Tomi
Meaning: Rich
Origin: Japanese

Tony/Toni
Meaning: Worthy of praise
Origin: Latin

Tonya
Meaning: Praiseworthy
Origin: Unknown

Trinika
Meaning: Pure
Origin: African American

Tyonna
Meaning: Princess
Origin: American

U

Udele
Meaning: Wealthy
Origin: English

Ukeme
Meaning: Ability, strength, skill
Origin: African

Uliana
Meaning: Youthful
Origin: Russian

Ulrika
Meaning: Prosperous
Origin: Scandinavian

Uma
Meaning: Tranquility
Origin: Indian

Uzuri
Meaning: Beauty
Origin: African

V

Varaidzo
Meaning: Entertainment
Origin: African-Zimbabwe

Velena
Meaning: Healthy
Origin: Latin

Veronica
Meaning: She who brings victory
Origin: Greek

Viveka
Meaning: Wisdom
Origin: Indian

W

Wakeisha
Meaning: Derived from Keisha meaning great joy
Origin: Jamaican

Willow
Meaning: Slender, graceful
Origin: English

Wincy
Meaning: Beautiful
Origin: English

Winola
Meaning: Gracious, charming friend
Origin: German

Wyanet
Meaning: Beautiful
Origin: American

X

Xarika
Meaning: Life blessing, princess
Origin: Arabic

Xenia
Meaning: Hospitable, welcoming
Origin: Greek

Xin
Meaning: Beautiful
Origin: Chinese

Y

Yafit
Meaning: Beautiful
Origin: Hebrew

Yakeera
Meaning: Beloved, precious
Origin: Hebrew

Yinka
Meaning: I am surrounded by wealth
Origin: African

Yori
Meaning: Reliable, trustworthy
Origin: Japanese

Z

Zadie
Meaning: Prosperous, fortunate
Origin: Arabic

Zahwa
Meaning: Joy, beauty, happiness
Origin: Arabic

Zaila
Meaning: Power
Origin: Arabic

Zana
Meaning: Wise
Origin: Kurdish

Zara
Meaning: Radiance
Origin: Arabic

Zareen
Meaning: Full of expression and smile
Origin: Arabic

Zeena
Meaning: Beautiful
Origin: African–Morocco

Zella
Meaning: Happy, blessed
Origin: Yiddish

Zen
Meaning: Meditation
Origin: Japanese

Zene
Meaning: Beautiful
Origin: African–Nigeria

Ziza
Meaning: Splendor, abundance
Origin: Hebrew

Zohar
Meaning: Brilliance
Origin: Hebrew

Zunaira
Meaning: Guiding light
Origin: Arabic

SPACE & NATURE

"Shoot for the moon. Even if you miss, you'll land in the stars."

Girl ♀

A

Abeba
Meaning: Flower
Origin: Ethiopian

Adama
Meaning: Earth
Origin: Hebrew

Alona
Meaning: Oak tree
Origin: Hebrew

Alondra
Meaning: Defender
Origin: Spanish

Amethyst
Meaning: Precious purple jewel
Origin: Greek

Amitola
Meaning: Rainbow
Origin: Native American

Arali
Meaning: The base of the Earth
Origin: Greek

Arden
Meaning: Great forest
Origin: Latin

Aurora
Meaning: Dawn
Origin: Latin

Avani
Meaning: Earth
Origin: Sanskrit

Awena
Meaning: Sunrise
Origin: Native American

B

Baca
Meaning: A mulberry tree
Origin: Biblical

Berkley
Meaning: Birch tree meadow
Origin: Old English

Blair
Meaning: Field, plain
Origin: Scottish

Blossom
Meaning: Flower like
Origin: English

Brook
Meaning: Water, stream
Origin: English

Brooke
Meaning: Brook, stream
Origin: English

Brooklyn
Meaning: Beautiful brook
Origin: English

C

Camellia
Meaning: Flower
Origin: Latin

Chamomile
Meaning: A fragrant herb
Origin: English

Chantrelle
Meaning: Stone
Origin: Old French

Charlene
Meaning: Free
Origin: German

Cinnamon
Meaning: A spice
Origin: Greek

Citali
Meaning: Star
Origin: Native American

Citana
Meaning: Star in the sky
Origin: Native American

Clover
Meaning: Flower
Origin: English

Coral
Meaning: Sea growth
Origin: Latin

Coraline
Meaning: Coral of the sea
Origin: American

Crystal
Meaning: Ice
Origin: Greek

D

Dahlia
Meaning: A flower
Origin: Scandinavian

Damani
Meaning: Tomorrow
Origin: American

Danica
Meaning: Morning star
Origin: Slavic

Daphne
Meaning: Laurel tree
Origin: Greek

Deborah
Meaning: Bee
Origin: Hebrew

Derry
Meaning: Oak grove
Origin: Irish

Diamond
Meaning: High value, brilliant
Origin: English

E

Ebony
Meaning: Black wood
Origin: English

Edana
Meaning: Fire
Origin: Gaelic

Ela
Meaning: Tree
Origin: Hebrew

Elara
Meaning: One of the moons of Jupiter
Origin: Greek

Elodie
Meaning: Marsh flower
Origin: Greek

Elon
Meaning: Oak tree
Origin: Hebrew

Elora
Meaning: Sun ray
Origin: Greek

Emerald
Meaning: Precious gemstone
Origin: Spanish

Ennis
Meaning: Island
Origin: Irish

Estelle
Meaning: Star
Origin: Unknown

Esther
Meaning: Star
Origin: Unknown

Evon
Meaning: Yew
Origin: French

F

Faviola
Meaning: Pink flower
Origin: Latin

Fawn
Meaning: Young deer
Origin: French

Fleur
Meaning: Flower
Origin: French

Flora
Meaning: Flower
Origin: Latin

Floressa
Meaning: Flower
Origin: Latin

Floretta
Meaning: Flower
Origin: Latin

Freesia
Meaning: A flower
Origin: Latin

G

Gaia
Meaning: Mother Earth
Origin: Greek

Galaxy
Meaning: Large system of stars
Origin: American

Gardenia
Meaning: Fragrant flower
Origin: English

Gemma
Meaning: Precious Stone
Origin: Italian

Geneva
Meaning: Juniper berry
Origin: Germanic

Georgia
Meaning: A girl who works the soil
Origin: Greek

Geranium
Meaning: Geranium flower
Origin: Greek

Greta
Meaning: Pearl
Origin: German

H

Halle
Meaning: Ruler, heroine
Origin: Scandinavian

Haracha
Meaning: Frog
Origin: African

Hayden
Meaning: Hay valley
Origin: English

Hibiscus
Meaning: A flower
Origin: Latin

Hyacinth
Meaning: Blue lapskur flower
Origin: Greek

Hyacinth
Meaning: A flower
Origin: Greek

I

Iara
Meaning: Water lady
Origin: Brazilian

India
Meaning: River
Origin: Unknown

Inika
Meaning: Small earth
Origin: Sanskrit

Ione
Meaning: Violet flower
Origin: Greek

Iris
Meaning: Rainbow
Origin: Greek

Isla
Meaning: Island
Origin: Scottish

Ixia
Meaning: South African flower
Origin: African

J

Jacintha
Meaning: Hyacinth
Origin: Dutch

Jasmina
Meaning: Jasmine flower
Origin: Persian

Jesenia
Meaning: Jasmine flower
Origin: Spanish

Juno
Meaning: Youth. Also a NASA space probe orbiting Jupiter
Origin: Latin

K

Kailani
Meaning: Sea and sky
Origin: Hawaiian

Kaito
Meaning: Ocean
Origin: Japanese

Kaleena
Meaning: A flower name
Origin: Slavic

Kalina
Meaning: Flower
Origin: Slavic

Kalinda
Meaning: The sun
Origin: Indian

Kalynda
Meaning: The sun
Origin: Indian

Kamaria
Meaning: Moonlight
Origin: Swahili

Kanika
Meaning: An atom, molecule
Origin: Indian

Kanoni
Meaning: Type of small bird
Origin: Swahili

Kenna
Meaning: Fire born
Origin: Gaelic

Kenya
Meaning: Country in Africa
Origin: Africa

Keziah
Meaning: Cassia tree
Origin: Hebrew

Kisha
Meaning: Rainfall
Origin: Slavic

Kishil
Meaning: Night
Origin: Native American

L

La-Verne
Meaning: Alder tree grove
Origin: French

Laila
Meaning: Night, dark
Origin: Arabic

Lake
Meaning: Body of water
Origin: British

Laurel
Meaning: Laurel tree
Origin: Latin

Lauren
Meaning: Laurel tree or laurel plant
Origin: French

Lavern
Meaning: Alder tree grove
Origin: French

Lavonne
Meaning: Wood
Origin: English

Leila
Meaning: Night
Origin: Arabic

Leilani
Meaning: Heavenly flower
Origin: Hawaiian

Lennox
Meaning: With many elm trees
Origin: Gaelic

Lesley
Meaning: Holly garden
Origin: English

Lila
Meaning: Night
Origin: Arabic

Liliana
Meaning: Lily, flower
Origin: Latin

Lorna
Meaning: The laurel tree
Origin: Scottish

Lumi
Meaning: Snow
Origin: Finnish

Luna
Meaning: Moon
Origin: Latin

Lyra
Meaning: A small constellation
Origin: Greek

M

Mae
Meaning: After the Roman Goddess of spring growth
Origin: Latin

Magnolia
Meaning: A flower
Origin: Latin

Mahina
Meaning: Moon
Origin: Hawaiian

Maletsasi
Meaning: Sunshine
Origin: African

Manuka
Meaning: Tree which produces honey
Origin: Sri Lanka

Mareena
Meaning: Of the sea
Origin: Latin

Maria
Meaning: Star of the sea
Origin: Latin

Marian
Meaning: Star of the sea, grace
Origin: French/Hebrew

Marietta
Meaning: Star of The Sea
Origin: French

Marisa
Meaning: Of the sea
Origin: Latin/Italian

Marjani
Meaning: Coral
Origin: African

Marley
Meaning: Lake meadow
Origin: English

Marlow
Meaning: Driftwood
Origin: British

Martinique

Meaning: Island in the Caribbean
Origin: French

Maurita

Meaning: Star of the sea
Origin: Latin

Meadow

Meaning: Field of grass
Origin: American

Meagan

Meaning: Pearl
Origin: Welsh

Meghan

Meaning: Pearl
Origin: Welsh

Moana

Meaning: Ocean, sea
Origin: Hawaiian

Moesha

Meaning: Drawn out of the water
Origin: Hebrew

Montana

Meaning: Mountain
Origin: Unknown

N

Nairobi

Meaning: Cool water
Origin: Unknown

Namazzi

Meaning: Water
Origin: Unknown

Nanala

Meaning: Sunflower
Origin: Hawaiian

Nash

Meaning: Dweller by the ash tree
Origin: English

Nerissa

Meaning: From the sea
Origin: Greek

Nisha

Meaning: Night
Origin: Indian

Nishay

Meaning: Night
Origin: Indian

North

Meaning: North
Origin: British

Nova
Meaning: New. Also, an astronomical event that causes the sudden appearance of light
Origin: Latin

Nyeleti
Meaning: Star
Origin: African

Nyeredzi
Meaning: Star
Origin: African

Nylah
Meaning: Cloud
Origin: Gaelic

Nyx
Meaning: Night
Origin: Greek

O

Ocean
Meaning: Sea
Origin: Greek

Oceana
Meaning: Ocean
Origin: Greek

Odina
Meaning: Mountain
Origin: Native American

Ohio
Meaning: Great river
Origin: Native American

Olivia
Meaning: Olive tree
Origin: Latin

Opal
Meaning: Gem
Origin: Sanskrit

Ornella
Meaning: Flowering ash tree
Origin: Italian/German

P

Paloma
Meaning: Dove
Origin: Spanish

Parker
Meaning: Keeper of the park
Origin: English

Peony
Meaning: Flower
Origin: Greek

Petunia
Meaning: Flower from nightshade family
Origin: English/Latin

Phillis
Meaning: Foliage
Origin: Greek

Phoenix
Meaning: Dark red
Origin: Greek

Primrose
Meaning: First rose
Origin: British

Q

Qamara
Meaning: The Moon
Origin: Arabic

Queisha
Meaning: Spice tree, cassia tree
Origin: African

R

Rai
Meaning: Thunder
Origin: Unknown

Rayen
Meaning: Flower
Origin: Native American

Rhea
Meaning: Flowing stream. Also, one of the moons of Saturn
Origin: Greek

Ria
Meaning: River
Origin: Spanish

Rio
Meaning: River
Origin: Spanish

River
Meaning: Stream of water that flows to the sea
Origin: English

Rocket

Meaning: A jet propelled tube
Origin: English

Romy

Meaning: Dew of the sea
Origin: Latin

Rosalyn

Meaning: Little rose
Origin: Spanish

Rosina

Meaning: Rose
Origin: Unknown

Ruby

Meaning: A deep red precious stone
Origin: Latin

S

Sabrina

Meaning: From the river (Severn)
Origin: Latin

Safari

Meaning: Journey
Origin: African

Saffron

Meaning: A yellow flower and spice
Origin: Arabic

Sahara

Meaning: Desert
Origin: Unknown

Sapphire

Meaning: Blue. Also a jewel and birthstone of September
Origin: Hebrew

Satima

Meaning: Young bull
Origin: African

Saturn

Meaning: The Roman God of wealth & agriculture. Also a ringed planet in our solar system
Origin: Latin

Savannah

Meaning: Treeless plain
Origin: Spanish

Sela

Meaning: Rock
Origin: Hebrew

Shakeia

Meaning: Hill
Origin: Unknown

Shareese/Sharise
Meaning: Grace
Origin: Greek

Shoshana
Meaning: Lily
Origin: Hebrew

Sidney
Meaning: Wide meadow
Origin: English

Sierra
Meaning: Mountain
Origin: Spanish

Solana
Meaning: Sunlight
Origin: Spanish

Soleil
Meaning: Sun
Origin: French

Star
Meaning: Luminous astronomical object
Origin: Greek

Stormy
Meaning: Impetuous nature
Origin: American

Summer
Meaning: Summer
Origin: Old English

Susie
Meaning: Lily
Origin: Hebrew

T

Takira
Meaning: Sun
Origin: American

Tamara/Tamera
Meaning: Date
Origin: Hebrew

Tanginika
Meaning: Lake Goddess
Origin: American

Tashina
Meaning: Beauty of the mountains
Origin: American

Tawanda
Meaning: Young tree
Origin: Zimbabwean

Tawni
Meaning: Green field
Origin: Irish

Tayen
Meaning: New moon
Origin: Native American

Taytu
Meaning: Sun
Origin: Amharic

Terra
Meaning: Earth
Origin: Latin

Thaba
Meaning: Mountain
Origin: African

Thuraia
Meaning: Star
Origin: Arabic

Tierra
Meaning: Earth
Origin: Spanish

Timber
Meaning: Wood
Origin: English

U

Usha
Meaning: Dawn
Origin: Indian

V

Varda
Meaning: Rose
Origin: Hebrew

Venus
Meaning: Roman Goddess of love. Also a planet in our solar system (2nd closest to the sun)
Origin: Greek

W

Wainani
Meaning: Beautiful water
Origin: Hawaiian

Willow
Meaning: Slender, graceful
Origin: English

Winter
Meaning: Cold season
Origin: American

Wren
Meaning: Small bird
Origin: English

X

Xia
Meaning: Glow of the sunrise
Origin: Chinese

Y

Yalissa
Meaning: A beautiful flower
Origin: Hebrew

Yalonda
Meaning: Violet flower
Origin: Spanish

Yevette/Yvette
Meaning: Yew tree
Origin: German/French

Yolande
Meaning: Purple
Origin: Latin

Z

Zabrina
Meaning: Fruitful desert flower
Origin: American

Zima
Meaning: Winter
Origin: Slavic

Zinnia
Meaning: Flower
Origin: Latin

Zola
Meaning: A lump of Earth
Origin: Latin

Zora
Meaning: Dawn
Origin: Arabic

Zorana
Meaning: Derived from Zora meaning dawn
Origin: Arabic

AFRICAN ORIGIN

"If we stand tall, it's because we stand on the shoulders of our ancestors." -African Proverb

Girl ♀

A

Ababuo
Meaning: A child that keeps coming back
Origin: African–Ghana

Abebi
Meaning: She came after asking
Origin: African–Nigeria

Abeje
Meaning: Asked For
Origin: African–Yoruba (Nigeria)

Abena
Meaning: Born on Tuesday
Origin: African–Ghana

Abiba
Meaning: The beloved one
Origin: Africa- North Africa

Abiola
Meaning: Born in honor /wealth
Origin: African–Nigeria

Abiona
Meaning: Born during a journey
Origin: African–Nigeria

Acanit
Meaning: Hard times
Origin: African–Uganda

Achen
Meaning: A girl twin
Origin: African–Uganda

Adanna
Meaning: Father's daughter
Origin: African- Igbo (Nigeria)

Adebayo
Meaning: Born in a joyful time
Origin: African

Adeniyi
Meaning: The crown has honor
Origin: African

Adhiambo
Meaning: Born after sunset
Origin: African

Adina
Meaning: She has saved
Origin: African

Adwoa
Meaning: Born on Monday
Origin: African- Ghana

Afafa
Meaning: First born child with a second husband
Origin: African–Ghana

Afia

Meaning: Born on Friday
Origin: African-Ghana

Afiya

Meaning: Healthy baby, free from illness
Origin: African

Africa

Meaning: From Africa
Origin: African

Afua

Meaning: Born on Friday
Origin: African

Afya

Meaning: Good health
Origin: African

Agbenyaga

Meaning: Life is precious
Origin: African-Ghana

Aissa

Meaning: Grateful
Origin: African

Ajua

Meaning: Born on Monday
Origin: African

Akande

Meaning: First born
Origin: African-Yoruba (Nigeria)

Akanke

Meaning: To know her is to love Her
Origin: African-Nigeria

Akello

Meaning: Child after twins
Origin: African-Uganda

Akinyi

Meaning: One who was born in morning
Origin: African

Akosua

Meaning: Born on Sunday
Origin: African-Ghana

Akua

Meaning: Born on Wednesday
Origin: African-Ghana

Alitash

Meaning: May I not lose you
Origin: African-Ethiopian

Alora

Meaning: My dream
Origin: African-Botswana

Ama

Meaning: Born on Saturday
Origin: African - Ghana

Amachi

Meaning: Gift from God
Origin: African-Zulu

Amadika
Meaning: Beloved
Origin: African–Kenya

Amalhe
Meaning: The beautiful one
Origin: African

Amandla
Meaning: Power
Origin: African–South Africa

Amondi
Meaning: Born at dawn
Origin: African–Ghana

Anana
Meaning: Soft, gentle
Origin: African–Ghana

Anashe
Meaning: Lord is with you
Origin: African

Anesu
Meaning: God is with us
Origin: African–Zimbabwe

Annakiya
Meaning: Sweet of face
Origin: African–Nigeria

Anuli
Meaning: Brings happiness
Origin: African–Nigeria

Anulika
Meaning: Happiness is the best
Origin: African–Nigeria

Apara
Meaning: A child who comes and goes
Origin: African–Nigeria

Arziki
Meaning: Prosperity
Origin: African

Asha
Meaning: Hope
Origin: African

Athiambo
Meaning: Born in the late evening
Origin: African

Audi
Meaning: Last daughter
Origin: African

Ayana
Meaning: Beautiful flower
Origin: African–Swahili

Ayira
Meaning: The chosen one
Origin: African

Ayo
Meaning: Happiness, joy
Origin: African- Nigeria

Ayoka
Meaning: One who causes joy
Origin: African

Azana
Meaning: Ultimate
Origin: African

Azinza
Meaning: Mermaid
Origin: African

Azmera
Meaning: Harvest
Origin: African

Azuka
Meaning: Support is paramount
Origin: African

B

Baako
Meaning: First born child
Origin: African

Baba
Meaning: Born on Thursday
Origin: African

Babirye
Meaning: Elder twin sister
Origin: luganda

Bacia
Meaning: Family death ruined the home
Origin: African–Uganda

Badu
Meaning: Tenth born
Origin: African–Ashanti of Ghana

Banji
Meaning: Second born twin
Origin: African

Barika
Meaning: Successful, blossom
Origin: African

Berhane
Meaning: My light
Origin: African–Ethiopia

Bibi
Meaning: Daughter of a king
Origin: African

Bina
Meaning: To sing, dance
Origin: African

Bisa
Meaning: Greatly loved
Origin: African

Bolade
Meaning: Honor arrives
Origin: African–Nigeria

Bunmi
Meaning: Gift
Origin: African

C

Caimile
Meaning: A family is born
Origin: African

Chalondra
Meaning: Smart
Origin: African

Chaonaine
Meaning: It has seen me
Origin: African

Chikelu
Meaning: Created by God
Origin: African

Chikere
Meaning: Created by God
Origin: African

Chinara
Meaning: May God receive
Origin: African–Nigeria

Chinue
Meaning: God's blessing
Origin: African–Nigeria

D

Dada
Meaning: Curly hair
Origin: African

Daia
Meaning: Everlasting morning
Origin: African

Damilola
Meaning: God has given me wealth
Origin: African

Dayo
Meaning: Happiness has come
Origin: African

Deka
Meaning: Pleasing
Origin: African

Delu
Meaning: The only girl
Origin: African

Dembe
Meaning: Peace
Origin: African

Dera
Meaning: Destiny
Origin: African

Desta
Meaning: Joy
Origin: African

Diara
Meaning: Gift
Origin: African

Dintle
Meaning: Beauty
Origin: African

Djenaba
Meaning: Affectionate
Origin: African

Douye
Meaning: Desire
Origin: African

Dumi
Meaning: The inspirer
Origin: African

Dziko
Meaning: Earth
Origin: African

E

Ebele
Meaning: Mercy, kindness
Origin: African

Ebere
Meaning: One who shows mercy
Origin: African

Eduwa
Meaning: This child is a messenger
Origin: African

Ekene
Meaning: Praise
Origin: African

Ellema
Meaning: Someone who milks a cow
Origin: African

Ellone
Meaning: God loves me
Origin: African

Eshe
Meaning: Life
Origin: African

Esi
Meaning: Born on a Sunday
Origin: African

Esiankiki
Meaning: Young maiden
Origin: African

Ezinwene
Meaning: Good brothers/ good sisters
Origin: African

F

Fabayo
Meaning: A lucky birth that gives joy
Origin: African

Fadzai
Meaning: Entertain, to make someone happy
Origin: African

Falala
Meaning: Born into abundance
Origin: African

Fana
Meaning: One who provides light
Origin: African

Fanta
Meaning: Beautiful day
Origin: African

Farai
Meaning: Rejoice, be happy
Origin: African

Fashola
Meaning: Makes wealth
Origin: African

Fayola
Meaning: Good fortune
Origin: African

Fola
Meaning: Honor
Origin: African

Folade
Meaning: Honor comes with this child
Origin: African

Folami
Meaning: Respect me
Origin: African

Folasade
Meaning: Honor earns a crown
Origin: African

G

Gamuchirai
Meaning: To receive
Origin: African

Genet
Meaning: Eden
Origin: African

Gimbya
Meaning: Princess
Origin: African

Gugu
Meaning: Precious
Origin: African

Gzifa
Meaning: Peaceful one
Origin: African

H

Haracha
Meaning: Frog
Origin: African

Hawa
Meaning: Desire
Origin: African

I

Ifama
Meaning: All is well
Origin: African

Ife
Meaning: Love
Origin: African

Ifeoma
Meaning: A good thing
Origin: African

Ifetayo
Meaning: Love brings happiness
Origin: African

Ifiok
Meaning: Wisdom
Origin: African

Isoke
Meaning: Satisfying gift from God
Origin: African

Isondo
Meaning: Wheel
Origin: African

Ixia
Meaning: South African flower
Origin: African

Izegbe
Meaning: The long-awaited child
Origin: African

J

Jaha
Meaning: Dignified
Origin: Swahili

Jahzara
Meaning: Blessed princess
Origin: African

Japera
Meaning: We have finished
Origin: African

Jendayi
Meaning: Grateful, thankful
Origin: African

Jendyose
Meaning: I have done good to produce this child
Origin: African

Jenue
Meaning: From Jenue in Nigeria
Origin: African

Jioni
Meaning: Evening
Origin: Swahili

Jira
Meaning: Related by blood
Origin: African

Jirani
Meaning: Neighbor
Origin: African-Swahili

Johari
Meaning: Gem, something of value
Origin: African-Swahili

Jokha
Meaning: Jeweled robe
Origin: African

Juji
Meaning: Heap of love
Origin: African

Jumapili
Meaning: Born on Sunday
Origin: African

Jumoke
Meaning: Everyone loves the child
Origin: African

K

Kabibe
Meaning: Little lady
Origin: African

Kacela
Meaning: A great huntress
Origin: African

Kagiso
Meaning: Peace
Origin: African

Kainda
Meaning: Hunter's daughter
Origin: African

Kamaria
Meaning: Moonlight
Origin: African–Swahili

Kambo
Meaning: Must work for everything
Origin: African

Kande
Meaning: Firstborn daughter
Origin: African

Kanene
Meaning: Little thing in the eye is big
Origin: African

Kapuki
Meaning: First born daughter
Origin: African

Karasi
Meaning: Full of life and wisdom
Origin: African

Karna
Meaning: Horn of an animal
Origin: African

Kasinda
Meaning: Born after twins
Origin: African

Katlego
Meaning: Success
Origin: African

Katleho
Meaning: Success
Origin: African

Kayin
Meaning: Long-awaited child
Origin: African

Keeya
Meaning: Garden flower
Origin: African

Keita
Meaning: Blessing
Origin: African

Kemi
Meaning: To be pampered
Origin: African

Kenya

Meaning: Country in Africa
Origin: Africa

Kenyatta

Meaning: Musician
Origin: African

Kerubo

Meaning: Born on the plain
Origin: African

Keshia

Meaning: Favorite
Origin: African

Kesi

Meaning: A child born when her father was in trouble
Origin: African

Keyah

Meaning: In good health
Origin: African

Kianga

Meaning: Sunshine
Origin: African

Kibibi

Meaning: Little lady
Origin: Swahili

Kiden

Meaning: Female born after 3+ boys
Origin: African

Kifimbo

Meaning: Very thin child
Origin: African

Kijana

Meaning: Youth
Origin: African

Kimani

Meaning: Adventurer
Origin: African

Kinaya

Meaning: Whole
Origin: African

Kione

Meaning: Someone who comes from nowhere
Origin: African

Kioni

Meaning: She who sees
Origin: African

Kirabo

Meaning: Gift from God
Origin: African

Kisembo

Meaning: Gift
Origin: African

Kissa

Meaning: First born daughter
Origin: African

Kitoko
Meaning: Beautiful
Origin: African

Kokumo
Meaning: This child will not die
Origin: African

Kuda
Meaning: God's intention
Origin: African

Kukua
Meaning: Born on a Wednesday
Origin: African

Kumani
Meaning: Destiny
Origin: African

Kwashi
Meaning: Born on Sunday
Origin: African

Kwayera
Meaning: Dawn
Origin: African

Kya
Meaning: Diamond in the sky
Origin: African

L

Lanecia
Meaning: Life
Origin: African–Swahili

Lela
Meaning: Black beauty
Origin: African

Lerato
Meaning: Song of my soul, to adore a person
Origin: African

Lewa
Meaning: Beautiful
Origin: African

Liseli
Meaning: Light
Origin: African

Lisimba
Meaning: Lion
Origin: African

Lulama
Meaning: The humble one
Origin: African

Lutendo
Meaning: Faith
Origin: African

M

Maame
Meaning: Mother
Origin: African

Mabinty
Meaning: Princess
Origin: African

Macia
Meaning: Orphan
Origin: African–Mozambique

Madea
Meaning: Matriarch of the family
Origin: African

Magara
Meaning: To sit, to stay
Origin: African

Mahari
Meaning: Forgiver
Origin: African

Maikulu
Meaning: Old mother
Origin: African

Maizah
Meaning: Discerning
Origin: African

Makadisa
Meaning: Good feeling towards
Origin: African

Makeba
Meaning: Greatness, precious jewel
Origin: African

Makeda
Meaning: Greatness. Also, the Ethiopic name for the Queen of Sheba
Origin: African

Makena
Meaning: Happy one
Origin: African

Makondo
Meaning: War
Origin: African

Malaika
Meaning: Angel
Origin: African

Maletsasi
Meaning: Sunshine
Origin: African

Mamello
Meaning: Patience
Origin: African

Mandisa
Meaning: Sweet
Origin: African

Manyara
Meaning: Humbled
Origin: African

Mariama
Meaning: Gift of God
Origin: African

Marjani
Meaning: Coral
Origin: African

Masani
Meaning: One with a gap between front teeth
Origin: African

Mashaka
Meaning: Trouble
Origin: African

Mashava
Meaning: Red
Origin: African–Zimbabwe

Masika
Meaning: Born during rain
Origin: African

Mawusi
Meaning: In the hands of God
Origin: African–Ghana

Mbalenhle
Meaning: Beautiful flower
Origin: African–Zulu

Mbeke
Meaning: Born at the beginning of the week
Origin: African

Melitte
Meaning: Full of grace
Origin: African

Mesi
Meaning: Water
Origin: African

Mhina
Meaning: Delightful
Origin: African–Bakongo of Zaire

Mikaili
Meaning: Who is like God?
Origin: African

Mikenna
Meaning: Who brings joy
Origin: African

Minana
Meaning: Miracle
Origin: African–Bantu of Zimbabwe

Miremba
Meaning: Promoter of peace
Origin: African

Miriro
Meaning: The one who was waited for
Origin: African–Shona

Miyanda
Meaning: Roots
Origin: African

Monifa
Meaning: Lucky
Origin: African–Egypt

Morowa
Meaning: Queen
Origin: African–Ghana

Msiba
Meaning: Born during calamity, misfortune
Origin: African–Swahili

Mufaro
Meaning: Happiness
Origin: African–Zimbabwe

Mugisa/Mugisha
Meaning: Blessing
Origin: African

Mwanawa
Meaning: First child
Origin: African

Mwasaa
Meaning: Well timed
Origin: African–Swahili

N

Naa
Meaning: Queen
Origin: African

Nabulungi
Meaning: Beautiful
Origin: African

Nacala
Meaning: Peace, tranquility
Origin: African–Lomwe of Mozambique

Nafula
Meaning: Born in the rainy season
Origin: African

Nafuna
Meaning: Delivered feet first
Origin: African

Nairobi
Meaning: Cool water
Origin: African

Nakato
Meaning: Second born of female twins
Origin: African

Nakimera
Meaning: Gift from God
Origin: African–Uganda

Nala
Meaning: Successful
Origin: African

Nalo
Meaning: Loveable
Origin: African

Namazzi
Meaning: Water
Origin: African

Namono
Meaning: Youngest twin
Origin: African

Nandi
Meaning: Sweet
Origin: African–Zulu

Nangila
Meaning: Born on a journey
Origin: African–Luya

Nanyamka
Meaning: God's gift
Origin: African–Ghana

Naserian
Meaning: The lucky one
Origin: African

Nathifa
Meaning: Clean, pure
Origin: African

Natine
Meaning: Of the Natine tribe
Origin: African

Nayo
Meaning: Joyful, having great joy
Origin: African–Yoruba

Ndidi
Meaning: Patience
Origin: African–Nigeria

Nekesa
Meaning: Born during the harvest
Origin: African

Ngendo
Meaning: Traveler
Origin: African–Kenya

Ngoni
Meaning: Mercy
Origin: African–Zimbabwe

Ngozi
Meaning: Blessing
Origin: African, Nigeria

Nia
Meaning: Purpose, goal
Origin: African–Swahili

Niara
Meaning: Utmost purpose
Origin: African–Swahili

Nimeesha
Meaning: Princess
Origin: African

Njeri
Meaning: Belongs to a warrior.
Origin: African–Kikuyu of Kenya

Nkechi
Meaning: Gift of God
Origin: African, Nigeria

Nneke
Meaning: Prominent mother
Origin: African–Nigeria

Nnena
Meaning: Paternal grandmother
Origin: African–Nigeria

Nokutenda
Meaning: By faith
Origin: African–Zimbabwe

Nomatha
Meaning: Big surprise
Origin: African

Nombeko
Meaning: Respect
Origin: African

Nombulelo
Meaning: Gratitude
Origin: African–Xhosa of South Africa

Nomusa
Meaning: Merciful
Origin: African

Noxolo
Meaning: Peaceful
Origin: African–South Africa

Nsombi
Meaning: Abundant joy
Origin: African

Nsomi
Meaning: Well behaved child
Origin: African

Nthati
Meaning: One to love me
Origin: African–Basotho

Ntsako
Meaning: Joy, happiness
Origin: African

Ntsumi
Meaning: Angel
Origin: African

Nyakio
Meaning: Hard working
Origin: African–Kikuyu of Kenya

Nyako
Meaning: Girl
Origin: African–Kenya

Nyaradzo
Meaning: Comfort
Origin: African

Nyarai
Meaning: Humble
Origin: African–Shona

Nyasha
Meaning: Merciful, kind-hearted
Origin: African

Nyeleti
Meaning: Star
Origin: African

Nyeredzi
Meaning: Star
Origin: African

Nzila
Meaning: Path, way
Origin: African–Tonga of Zambia

Nzinga
Meaning: Beloved person who came from river
Origin: African

O

Oafe
Meaning: Your descent matters
Origin: African–Ishan of Nigeria

Obioma
Meaning: Kind-hearted
Origin: African–Nigeria

Ogochukwu
Meaning: The favor of God
Origin: African–Nigeria

Okal
Meaning: To cross
Origin: African

Okoth
Meaning: Born when it was raining
Origin: African

Olabisi
Meaning: Joy and honor have increased
Origin: African–Nigeria

Olabunmi
Meaning: Gift of God
Origin: African–Nigeria

Olajuwon
Meaning: Wealth and honor are God's gifts
Origin: African–Nigeria

Olushola
Meaning: God has blessed or honored me
Origin: African–Nigeria

Omarosa
Meaning: My precious and beautiful child
Origin: African–Nigeria

Omodara
Meaning: The child is Good
Origin: African–Nigeria

Omorose
Meaning: Beautiful
Origin: African

Omosede
Meaning: A child is more valuable than a king
Origin: African

Onaedo
Meaning: Gold
Origin: African–Nigeria

Oni
Meaning: Born on a sacred ground
Origin: African–Nigeria

Onyeka
Meaning: God is the greatest
Origin: African–Nigeria

Oraefo
Meaning: Affectionate
Origin: African

Oratilwe
Meaning: Loved one
Origin: African

Orma
Meaning: Free men
Origin: African–Kenya

Oseye
Meaning: One who is happy
Origin: African

P

Palesa
Meaning: Flower
Origin: African–Basotho of Lesotho

Panashe
Meaning: Where God is
Origin: African

Panyin
Meaning: Older of twins
Origin: African-Ghana

Pasua
Meaning: Born by cesarean
Origin: African-Swahili

Pedzi
Meaning: To finish
Origin: African

Pemba
Meaning: The force of present existence
Origin: African

Penda
Meaning: Love
Origin: African-Swahili

Phenyo
Meaning: Victory
Origin: African-Botswana

Puleng
Meaning: Out in the rain
Origin: African-Basotho

Q

Qalhata
Meaning: An Egyptian queen
Origin: African

Queisha
Meaning: Spice tree
Origin: African

Qwara
Meaning: An Ethiopian tribe name
Origin: African

R

Rafiki
Meaning: Friend
Origin: African-Kiswahili

Ramla
Meaning: Prophetess
Origin: African-Swahili

Rasida
Meaning: Rightly guided, righteous
Origin: African

Rudo
Meaning: Love
Origin: African–Zimbabwe

Rufaro
Meaning: Happiness
Origin: African–Zimbabwe

Runyararo
Meaning: Peace
Origin: African–Zimbabwe

Russom
Meaning: One who is a leader
Origin: African–Swahili

Rutendo
Meaning: Faith
Origin: African–Zimbabwe

Ruvarashe
Meaning: God's flower
Origin: African–Zimbabwe

Ruvimbo
Meaning: Faith
Origin: African–Zimbabwe

S

Sade
Meaning: Honor earns a crown
Origin: African

Safara
Meaning: Fire
Origin: African

Safari
Meaning: Journey
Origin: African

Saidi
Meaning: Helper
Origin: African

Samora
Meaning: Guarded by God
Origin: African

Sandile
Meaning: You have increased our family
Origin: African

Sanyu
Meaning: Happiness
Origin: African

Saran
Meaning: Joy
Origin: African

Sarki
Meaning: Chief
Origin: African

Sarudzai
Meaning: The chosen one
Origin: African

Satima
Meaning: Young bull
Origin: African

Sekai
Meaning: One who brings laughter and great joy
Origin: African

Sekelaga
Meaning: Rejoice
Origin: African

Selam
Meaning: Peace
Origin: African

Selasi
Meaning: God hears me
Origin: African

Serwa
Meaning: Noblewoman
Origin: African

Shamiso
Meaning: Miracle
Origin: African

Shandu
Meaning: Change
Origin: African

Shaniece
Meaning: Gift of God
Origin: African

Shantewa
Meaning: God's present
Origin: African

Shardea
Meaning: Honor earns the crown
Origin: African

Shasa
Meaning: Precious water
Origin: African

Shasmecka
Meaning: Princess
Origin: African

Shukura
Meaning: Grateful
Origin: African–Egypt

Sidone
Meaning: It is heard (like a prayer)
Origin: African

Sika
Meaning: Money
Origin: African

Siphiwe
Meaning: We were given
Origin: African

Sisi
Meaning: Born on Sunday
Origin: African

Siyanda
Meaning: We are growing
Origin: African

Sondo
Meaning: Born on Sunday
Origin: African

Ssanyu
Meaning: Joy
Origin: African

Subria
Meaning: Patience
Origin: African

Sukutai
Meaning: Hug
Origin: African

Syandene
Meaning: Punctual
Origin: African

T

Tabia
Meaning: Talented
Origin: African

Taifa
Meaning: Nation
Origin: African

Taiwo
Meaning: First twin to taste the world
Origin: African

Takunda
Meaning: We have overcome
Origin: African

Tamasha
Meaning: Pageant, show
Origin: African–Swahili

Tanasha
Meaning: Reigning queen
Origin: African

Tapanga
Meaning: Sweet
Origin: African

Taraji
Meaning: Hope
Origin: African

Tariro
Meaning: Hope
Origin: African

Tarisai
Meaning: Behold
Origin: African

Tawanda
Meaning: Young tree
Origin: Zimbabwean

Tendai
Meaning: Be thankful to God
Origin: African

Tendani
Meaning: Give thanks
Origin: African

Tene
Meaning: One who is much loved
Origin: African

Terehasa
Meaning: Blessed
Origin: African

Teshi
Meaning: Cheerful
Origin: African

Thaba
Meaning: Mountain
Origin: African

Thandiwe
Meaning: Beloved
Origin: African

Thema
Meaning: Queen
Origin: African

Tinashe
Meaning: God is with us
Origin: African

Tiombe
Meaning: Shy
Origin: African

Titilayo
Meaning: Eternal happiness
Origin: African

Tiwa
Meaning: One who owns the crown
Origin: African

U

Ubanwa
Meaning: The wealth of children
Origin: African

Uchechuckwu
Meaning: God's will
Origin: African

Udoka
Meaning: Peace is the greatest
Origin: African

Ukeme
Meaning: Ability, strength, skill
Origin: African

Usoa
Meaning: Dove
Origin: African

Uwimana
Meaning: Daughter of God
Origin: African

Uzuri
Meaning: Beauty
Origin: African

V

Varaidzo
Meaning: Entertainment
Origin: African–Zimbabwe

Venda
Meaning: Of the Bantu people
Origin: African–South Africa

Vimbai
Meaning: Have faith
Origin: African–Zimbabwe

Visola
Meaning: Longings are waterfalls
Origin: African

Visolela
Meaning: To use one's judgment
Origin: African

Vuyo
Meaning: Happiness
Origin: African–South Africa

W

Walta
Meaning: Shield
Origin: African–Kenya

Wangari
Meaning: A leopard
Origin: African–Kenya

Wawira
Meaning: Worker
Origin: African

Wesesa
Meaning: Careless
Origin: African

Winta

Meaning: Desire
Origin: African

X

Xetsa

Meaning: Twin
Origin: African

Xhosa

Meaning: Sweet. Also an official language of South Africa and Zimbabwe.
Origin: African–South Africa

Xola

Meaning: Stay in peace
Origin: African–Xhosa of South Africa

Xolani

Meaning: Stay in peace
Origin: African–Xhosa of South Africa

Y

Yaa

Meaning: Born on Thursday
Origin: African

Yassah

Meaning: A dance
Origin: African

Yejide

Meaning: Looks like her mother
Origin: African–Nigeria

Yenge

Meaning: Work
Origin: African–Mende of Sierra Leone

Yetunde

Meaning: Mother has returned
Origin: African–Yoruba

Yewubdar

Meaning: Beautiful beyond limits
Origin: African

Yihana

Meaning: Congratulations
Origin: African

Yinka

Meaning: I am surrounded by wealth
Origin: African

Yobachi
Meaning: Pray to God
Origin: African

Yohance
Meaning: God's gift
Origin: African

Z

Zaci
Meaning: God of fatherhood
Origin: African

Zaire
Meaning: The river that swallows other rivers
Origin: African

Zalika
Meaning: Well born
Origin: African–Swahili

Zanta
Meaning: Beautiful girl
Origin: African

Zawadi
Meaning: Gift
Origin: African–Swahili

Zendaya
Meaning: Be thankful
Origin: African–Bantu of Zimbabwe

Zene
Meaning: Beautiful
Origin: African–Nigeria

Zhenga
Meaning: African queen
Origin: African–South Africa

Zinhle
Meaning: Beautiful
Origin: African–Zulu

Ziraili
Meaning: Help of God
Origin: African

Zo
Meaning: Spiritual leader
Origin: African

Zoan
Meaning: Departure
Origin: African

Zufan
Meaning: Throne
Origin: African

Zuna
Meaning: To be sweet
Origin: African

Zuri

Meaning: Beautiful
Origin: African

Zuwena

Meaning: Good
Origin: African-Swahili

Zweena

Meaning: Beautiful
Origin: African-Morocco

BIBLICAL

"A good name is more to be desired than great wealth." –Proverbs 22:1

Girl ♀

A

Abana
Meaning: Made of stone
Origin: Hebrew

Abi
Meaning: My father is exalted
Origin: Hebrew

Abiah
Meaning: The Lord is my father
Origin: Hebrew

Adah
Meaning: Adornment
Origin: Hebrew

Adalia
Meaning: Noble one
Origin: Hebrew

Adaliah
Meaning: One that draws water
Origin: Hebrew

Addi
Meaning: Adorned
Origin: Unknown

Adna
Meaning: Pleasure, delight
Origin: Unknown

Adriel
Meaning: The flock of God
Origin: Hebrew

Asia
Meaning: Sunrise
Origin: Hebrew

B

Baca
Meaning: A mulberry tree
Origin: Hebrew

Bathsheba
Meaning: Daughter of the oath
Origin: Hebrew

Bethany
Meaning: House of figs. Also a town close to Jerusalem
Origin: Hebrew

Bethel
Meaning: House of God
Origin: Hebrew

C

Calah
Meaning: Opportunity
Origin: Arabic

Candace
Meaning: Pure
Origin: Latin

Chebar
Meaning: Force or strength
Origin: Biblical

Cleophas
Meaning: The whole glory
Origin: Latin

D

Dalaiah
Meaning: The poor of the Lord
Origin: Hebrew

Damaris
Meaning: Gentle
Origin: Greek

Daniella
Meaning: God is my judge
Origin: Hebrew

Dannah
Meaning: Judging
Origin: Hebrew

Darah
Meaning: Pearl of wisdom
Origin: Hebrew

Deborah
Meaning: Bee
Origin: Hebrew

Delilah
Meaning: Delicate, weakening
Origin: Hebrew

E

Eden
Meaning: Place of pleasure
Origin: Hebrew

Elizabeth
Meaning: God is my oath
Origin: Hebrew

Esther
Meaning: Star
Origin: Persian

Eunice
Meaning: Good victory
Origin: Greek

Eve
Meaning: To breathe, live
Origin: Hebrew

G

Gabriela
Meaning: God is my strength
Origin: Hebrew

Genesis
Meaning: The beginning
Origin: Greek

Gianna
Meaning: The Lord is gracious
Origin: Italian

H

Hadassah
Meaning: Myrtle tree
Origin: Hebrew

Hannah
Meaning: God has favored
Origin: Hebrew

Harran
Meaning: A singing
Origin: Hebrew

I

Iram
Meaning: Shining
Origin: Arabic

Iscah
Meaning: To behold
Origin: Hebrew

Israel
Meaning: May God prevail
Origin: Unknown

J

Jemima
Meaning: Dove
Origin: Hebrew

Jemimah
Meaning: Dove
Origin: Hebrew

Jesse
Meaning: The Lord exists
Origin: Hebrew

Joanna
Meaning: God is gracious
Origin: Hebrew

K

Keturah
Meaning: Fragrance
Origin: Hebrew

Kezia
Meaning: Cassia tree
Origin: Hebrew

Keziah
Meaning: Cassia tree
Origin: Hebrew

L

Lael
Meaning: Belonging to God
Origin: Hebrew

Leah
Meaning: Weary
Origin: Hebrew

Lois
Meaning: Most desirable
Origin: Greek

M

Makeda
Meaning: Greatness. Also, the Ethiopic name for the Queen of Sheba
Origin: African

Mary
Meaning: Beloved
Origin: Hebrew

N

Nehushta
Meaning: Made of brass
Origin: Hebrew

Neriah
Meaning: Lamp of the Lord
Origin: Hebrew

Nethaniah
Meaning: Given of Jehovah
Origin: Hebrew

O

Olive
Meaning: Fruitfulness, olive tree
Origin: Latin

Ophrah
Meaning: Fawn
Origin: Hebrew

P

Paula
Meaning: Small, humble
Origin: Latin

Phoebe
Meaning: Shining
Origin: Greek

Phoenicia
Meaning: Red/purple
Origin: Israel

Prisca
Meaning: Ancient
Origin: Latin

R

Rachel
Meaning: Ewe
Origin: Hebrew

Rebecca
Meaning: To bind
Origin: Hebrew

Rebekah
Meaning: Captivating
Origin: Hebrew

Ruth
Meaning: Compassionate friend
Origin: Hebrew

S

Samaria
Meaning: A watch tower
Origin: Hebrew

Sansannah
Meaning: Bough or bramble of the enemy
Origin: Biblical

Saphir
Meaning: Sapphire, gem
Origin: Biblical

Sapphira
Meaning: Sapphire, gem
Origin: Biblical

Sarah
Meaning: Noblewoman, princess
Origin: Hebrew

Sarai
Meaning: My lady, princess
Origin: Hebrew

Sela
Meaning: Rock
Origin: Hebrew

Shiloh
Meaning: Tranquil
Origin: Hebrew

Shiphrah
Meaning: Beautiful
Origin: Hebrew

T

Tabitha
Meaning: Gazelle
Origin: Aramaic

Talitha
Meaning: Little girl
Origin: Aramaic

Tamah
Meaning: Innocent, honest
Origin: Hebrew

Tanach
Meaning: Who humbles you
Origin: Biblical

Tirzah
Meaning: Delight
Origin: Hebrew

Z

Zanoah
Meaning: Forgetfulness
Origin: Hebrew

Zarah
Meaning: Shining, radiance
Origin: Biblical

Zaza
Meaning: Plenty, abundance
Origin: Biblical

Zemira
Meaning: Song
Origin: Hebrew

Zenas
Meaning: Hospitable
Origin: Greek

Ziha
Meaning: Brightness
Origin: Biblical

Zina
Meaning: Shining
Origin: Greek

Zipporah
Meaning: Bird
Origin: Hebrew

Ziza
Meaning: Splendor, abundance
Origin: Biblical/Hebrew

Zohar
Meaning: Brilliance
Origin: Hebrew

INFLUENTIAL PEOPLE

"I don't know who you will be but I know you will be my everything."

Girl ♀

A

Afeni

Meaning: Health
Origin: Arabic
Influential Person: Afeni Shakur – Political activist and mother of rapper, Tupac Shakur.

Alexa

Meaning: Defender of mankind
Origin: Greek
Influential Person: Alexa Canady – The first Black female Neurosurgeon in the USA.

Alice

Meaning: Noble
Origin: Greek
Influential Person: Alice Walker – Award-winning author and Pulitzer Prize Winner.

Allyson

Meaning: Noble
Origin: German
Influential Person: Alyson Felix – Multi Olympic medallist and one of Time Magazine's Most Influential People in 2020 and 2021

Althea

Meaning: Healer
Origin: Greek
Influential Person: Althea Gibson – First Black woman to win Wimbledon (tennis). She won 11 Grand Slam titles in her career.

Amanda

Meaning: Lovable
Origin: Greek
Influential Person: Amanda Gorman – Youngest inaugural poet in US history.

Amina

Meaning: Honest, faithful
Origin: Arabic
Influential Person: Queen Amina of Zazzau – A skilled military leader from the state of Zazzau (in modern-day Nigeria).

Angela

Meaning: Heavenly messenger
Origin: Greek
Influential Person: Angela Davis – Civil rights activist.

Annie

Meaning: Derived from Hannah meaning favor/grace
Origin: Hebrew
Influential Person: Annie Easley - Computer Scientist, Mathematician, Rocket Scientist, she worked at NASA as a "human computer".

Aubrey

Meaning: Ruler of The Elves, wise
Origin: French
Influential Person: Aubrey Graham aka Drake - Grammy award-winning rapper, actor, and entrepreneur.

Augusta

Meaning: Great, magnificent
Origin: Latin
Influential Person: Augusta Savage - American sculptor.

B

Beyoncé

Meaning: Beyond others
Origin: Creole
Influential Person: Beyonce Knowles - Grammy award-winning artist and one of the best-selling artists of all time with over 118m sold worldwide (as of 2021).

Bobby/Bobbie

Meaning: Famous, bright
Origin: German
Influential Person: Bobbie Brown - Grammy award-winning singer and rapper. Bobby Marshall - First Black footballer in the NFL (along with Fritz Pollard)

Brandy

Meaning: Warm and comforting
Origin: American
Influential Person: Brandy Norwood – Award-winning singer, songwriter, and actress.

C

Charlotte

Meaning: Free
Origin: French
Influential Person: Queen Charlotte of Britain – Allegedly the first Black royal in Britain.

Chloe

Meaning: Blooming
Origin: Greek
Influential Person: Chloe Bailey – Award-winning singer, songwriter, and actress.

Ciara

Meaning: Dark-haired
Origin: Irish
Influential Person: Ciara – Singer, songwriter, and model.

Claudia

Meaning: Lame
Origin: Latin
Influential Person: Claudia Jones – Founder of the UK's first major Black newspaper and one of the founders of Notting Hill Carnival.

Condoleeza

Meaning: With sweetness
Origin: Italian
Influential Person: Condoleeza Rice – Former US Secretary of State and first Black woman to hold the position.

D

Diana

Meaning: Divine
Origin: Greek
Influential Person: Diana Ross – Grammy award-winning artist and one of Motown's most successful artists of the 1960s.

Diane

Meaning: Divine
Origin: Latin
Influential Person: Diane Abbott – First Black woman to be elected to the UK parliament and the longest-serving Black MP in the House of Commons (as of 2021).

Dina

Meaning: Fair, judged
Origin: Hebrew
Influential Person: Dina Asher-Smith – Olympic bronze medallist and the fastest British woman in recorded history (at time of writing).

Doris

Meaning: Gift
Origin: Greek
Influential Person: Doris Miller – The first Black American to be awarded the Navy Cross.

E

Eartha

Meaning: Worldly/Earth
Origin: English
Influential Person: Earth Kitt – American Singer, actress & activist.

Elaine

Meaning: Torch of light
Origin: Greek
Influential Person: Elaine Thompson-Herah – 5-time Olympic champion and fastest woman in the World (as of 2021).

Ellen

Meaning: Shining light
Origin: Greek
Influential Person: Ellen Johnson Sirleaf – The first woman to become a head of state in Africa.

Etta

Meaning: Keeper of the hearth
Origin: French
Influential Person: Etta James – Grammy award-winning singer.

Eva

Meaning: Life
Origin: Hebrew
Influential Person: Eva Marcille – American Model, actress & previous winner of America's Top Model.

G

Gayle

Meaning: Father's joy
Origin: Hebrew
Influential Person: Gayle King – American TV personality, author, and broadcast journalist.

Gianna

Meaning: The Lord is gracious
Origin: Italian
Influential Person: Gianna Bryant – Young basketballer and daughter of Kobe Bryant.

Gwendolyn

Meaning: Blessed
Origin: Welsh
Influential Person: Gwendolyn Brooks – First Black author to win the Pulitzer Prize.

H

Halle

Meaning: Ruler, heroine
Origin: Scandinavian
Influential Person: Halle Berry – Academy Award-winning American actress and the first Black woman to win the Academy Award for Best Actress.

Harriet

Meaning: Home ruler
Origin: English
Influential Person: Harriet Tubman – Born into slavery, she escaped and went on to go back and rescue many slaves via the Underground Railroad. She was the first woman to lead an armed expedition in the American Civil War, where she liberated more than 700 enslaved people.

I

Issa

Meaning: Jesus
Origin: Arabic
Influential Person: Issa Rae – Award-winning actress, writer, and producer.

Ivy

Meaning: Faithfulness
Origin: English
Influential Person: Blue Ivy Carter – The second youngest person to win a Grammy award and youngest to win a BET award (as of 2021). She is the daughter of Beyonce & Jay-Z.

J

Jack

Meaning: Likely derived from the name John meaning God is gracious
Origin: Hebrew
Influential Person: Jack Johnson – First Black boxing heavyweight champion of the world.

Jackie

Meaning: Likely derived from the name John meaning God is gracious
Origin: Hebrew
Influential Person: Jackie Robinson – First Black player in Major League Baseball, winner of the National League Most Valuable Player award, and civil rights activist.

Jaden

Meaning: God has heard
Origin: Hebrew
Influential Person: Jaden Smith – American rapper and actor. Son of Will Smith and Jada Pinkett-Smith.

Janelle

Meaning: God is merciful
Origin: Hebrew
Influential Person: Janelle Monae – Award-winning singer, rapper, and actress.

Jennifer

Meaning: Fair one
Origin: Cornish
Influential Person: Jennifer Hudson – Academy Award and Grammy award-winning actress and singer.

Jesse

Meaning: The Lord exists
Origin: Hebrew
Influential Person: Jesse Owens – 4 times Olympic gold medallist and the most successful athlete at the 1936 Berlin Olympics (held in Germany when under Hitler's rule).

Joe

Meaning: God will give
Origin: Hebrew
Influential Person: Joe Louis – Professional boxer who is widely regarded as one of the best and most influential of all time.

Jordan

Meaning: Flowing down
Origin: Hebrew
Influential Person: Jordan Peele – Actor, comedian, and filmmaker. He was the first Black director to win an Academy Award for Best Original Screenplay.

K

Kamala

Meaning: Lotus flower
Origin: Indian
Influential Person: Kamala Harris – US Vice President and the first Black/first female to take the office.

Kara

Meaning: Beloved
Origin: Italian
Influential Person: Kara Walker – American artist, filmmaker, and professor.

Katherine

Meaning: Pure
Origin: Greek
Influential Person: Katherine Johnson – Mathematician. Her work helped put the first US astronaut in space and the first-ever humans on the moon.

Kyrie

Meaning: Lord
Origin: Greek
Influential Person: Kyrie Irving – American basketballer.

L

Latoya

Meaning: Victorious one
Origin: Spanish
Influential Person: Latoyah Luckett – Former member of the award-winning band Destiny's Child.

Lennox

Meaning: With many elm trees
Origin: Gaelic
Influential Person: Lennox Lewis – British former heavyweight boxing champion of the world.

M

Madea

Meaning: Matriarch of the family
Origin: African
Influential Person: Madea Simmons – Popular character created by Tyler Perry.

Mae

Meaning: After the Roman Goddess of spring growth
Origin: Latin
Influential Person: Mae Jemison – Engineer, physician, and the first Black American woman to travel into space.

Magic

Meaning: Full of wonder
Origin: American
Influential Person: Earvin "Magic" Johnson – American professional basketball player who is widely considered the best point guard of all time.

Malorie

Meaning: Unfortunate
Origin: French
Influential Person: Malorie Blackman – Best-selling author and the first Black Children's Laureate.

Mari

Meaning: Star of the sea
Origin: Welsh
Influential Person: Mari Copeny – At just 8 years old she became a key figure in raising awareness of the Flint, Michigan water crisis.

Marian

Meaning: Star of the sea, grace
Origin: French/Hebrew
Influcntial Person: Marian Anderson – American contralto (classical singer) and a key figure in the effort to overcome racial prejudice in the USA in the mid-20th century.

Marie

Meaning: Star of the sea
Origin: Latin
Influential Person: Marie M. Daly – The first Black woman to receive a Ph.D. in Chemistry in the USA.

Marley

Meaning: Lake meadow
Origin: English
Influential Person: Marley Dias – Creator of the #1000BlackGirlsBooks–a movement calling for more books with Black girls as lead characters. The campaign led to the donation of 10s of 1000s of books and more publishers publishing books written by or featuring Black girls.

Marsha

Meaning: Warlike
Origin: Latin
Influential Person: Marsha P Johnson – Influential gay rights activist and a prominent figure in the Stonewall Uprisings.

Mary

Meaning: Beloved
Origin: Hebrew
Influential Person: Mary J. Blige – Grammy award-winning artist. Mary Seacole – Jamaican-born nurse who set up "The British Hotel" behind the lines in the Crimean War to care for wounded soldiers.

Maya

Meaning: Water
Origin: Hebrew
Influential Person: Maya Angelou – American civil rights activist, author, screenwriter, and award-winning poet.

Meghan

Meaning: Pearl
Origin: Welsh
Influential Person: Meghan Markle – Actress and member of the British Royal Family.

Meta

Meaning: Pearl
Origin: Greek
Influential Person: Meta Vaux Warrick Fuller – Poet, painter, theater designer, and sculptor of the Black American experience.

Michelle

Meaning: Who is like God?
Origin: French
Influential Person: Michelle Obama – An attorney, author & former First Lady of the USA.

Misty

Meaning: Covered with mist, dew
Origin: English
Influential Person: Misty Copeland – Ballet dancer and first Black woman to be made Principal Dancer in the American Ballet Theater's history.

Monique

Meaning: Advisor
Origin: French
Influential Person: Monique "Mo'nique" Hicks – Bafta award-winning actress and comedian.

Morgan

Meaning: Sea
Origin: Welsh
Influential Person: Morgan Freeman – Academy Award-winning actor.

N

Naomi

Meaning: Pleasantness
Origin: Hebrew
Influential Person: Naomi Campbell – British Supermodel. The first Black woman to appear on the cover of French Vogue and the first Black model on the cover of Time.

Neo/Neyo

Meaning: Gift
Origin: African Origin/American
Influential Person: Ne-Yo (Shaffer Smith) – Grammy Award-winning singer and songwriter.

Ngozi

Meaning: Blessing
Origin: African – Nigerian
Influential Person: Ngozi Okonjo-Iweala – Nigerian-American economist, fair trade leader, and current Director-General of the World Trade Organization (2021).

Nia

Meaning: Purpose, goal
Origin: Swahili
Influential Person: Nia Long – Award-winning American actress.

Nikki

Meaning: Victory of the people
Origin: American
Influential Person: Nikki Minaj (Onika Maraj-Petty) – Trinidad-born award-winning rapper. She is one of the best-selling female artists of all time with over 100m records sold worldwide.

Nina

Meaning: Favor, grace
Origin: Hebrew
Influential Person: Nina Simone – Award-winning singer, songwriter, and civil rights activist. She was inducted into the Grammy Hall of Fame in 2000.

Nzinga

Meaning: Beloved person who came from a river
Origin: African
Influential Person: Queen Nzinga Mbandi – Ruler of the kingdoms of Ndongo and Matamba (modern-day Angola).

O

Octavia

Meaning: Eighth
Origin: Latin
Influential Person: Octavia Lenora Spencer – Academy Award-winning American actress, author, and producer.

Onika

Meaning: A courageous soldier
Origin: Sanskrit
Influential Person: Onika Maraj-Petty aka Nikki Minaj – Trinidad-born award-winning rapper. She is one of the best-selling female artists of all time with over 100m records sold worldwide.

Oprah

Meaning: Derived from Orpah meaning gazelle, young deer, fawn
Origin: Hebrew
Influential Person: Oprah Winfrey – American TV host, producer, and philanthropist. Oprah was the first Black female billionaire.

P

Phillis

Meaning: Foliage
Origin: Greek
Influential Person: Phillis Wheatley – Sold into slavery, Phillis became a poet and the first Black woman to have a poem published.

R

Raven

Meaning: Dark-haired, wise
Origin: English
Influential Person: Raven Symone – Award-winning actress, singer, and songwriter.

Rebecca

Meaning: To bind
Origin: Hebrew
Influential Person: Rebecca Lee Crumpler – The first African American woman to qualify as a doctor.

Rihanna

Meaning: Great queen
Origin: Irish
Influential Person: Rihanna – Grammy award-winning singer, actress, fashion designer, and businesswoman. She is the wealthiest female musician (worth 1.7B as of 2021).

Rosa

Meaning: Rose
Origin: Spanish
Influential Person: Rosa Parks – Her refusal to give up her seat on a bus sparked the Montgomery Bus Boycott and the eventual Supreme Court decision to integrate the bus system there. Parks was a lifelong campaigner for civil rights causes.

Ruby

Meaning: A deep red precious stone
Origin: Latin
Influential Person: Ruby Bridges – The first Black student to attend the all-White William Frantz Elementary school at the height of desegregation.

Rumi

Meaning: Beauty
Origin: Japanese
Influential Person: Rumi Carter – Daughter of Beyonce Knowles & Jay Z.

S

Sade

Meaning: Honor earns a crown
Origin: African
Influential Person: Sade Adu – An award-winning singer and songwriter and the first Nigerian person to win a Grammy.

Sadie

Meaning: Princess
Origin: Hebrew
Influential Person: Sadie Tanner Mossell Alexander – American Lawyer, civil rights activist, and the first African American to receive a Ph.D. in economics in the US. She was the first African American woman to practice law in Pennsylvania.

Sanya

Meaning: Brilliant
Origin: Arabic
Influential Person: Sanya Richards-Ross – Jamaican-American Olympic gold medallist and the first American woman to win two global titles in the 400m.

Sarah

Meaning: Noblewoman, princess
Origin: Hebrew
Influential Person: Sarah Breedlove aka Madam CJ Walker – Inventor and entrepreneur; she was the first female self-made millionaire in the USA.

Sarah Jane Woodson Early – The first African American woman to teach at a university.

Sarah Boone – Pioneering inventor and inventor of the modern-day ironing board.

Serena

Meaning: Tranquil
Origin: Latin
Influential Person: Serena Williams – One of the most decorated female tennis players in history.

Shirley

Meaning: Bright meadow
Origin: English
Influential Person: Shirley Chisholm – First Black woman to be elected to Congress in the USA.

Shirley Bassey – British award-winning singer, famous for her James Bond themes "Goldfinger" and "Diamonds Are Forever".

Shonda

Meaning: God is gracious
Origin: American
Influential Person: Shonda Rhimes – Award-winning producer, screenwriter, and author.

Sidney

Meaning: Wide meadow
Origin: English
Influential Person: Sidney Poitier – The first Black actor to win an Academy Award.

Simone

Meaning: God has heard
Origin: Hebrew
Influential Person: Simone Biles – Artistic gymnast and (jointly) the most decorated gymnast of all time (as of 2021).

Sojourner

Meaning: To stay a while
Origin: English
Influential Person: Sojourner Truth – An abolitionist and women's rights activist. After going to court to recover her son in 1828, she became the first Black woman to win such a case against a white man.

Susie

Meaning: Lily
Origin: Hebrew
Influential Person: Susie Taylor – The first African American army nurse. She was never paid for her work.

T

Taraji

Meaning: Hope
Origin: African
Influential Person: Taraji P. Henson – Award-winning actress and the first Black woman to win a Critic's Choice Award For Best Actress in a Drama Series.

Taytu

Meaning: Sun
Origin: Amharic
Influential Person: Taytu Betul – Empress of Ethiopia, she established and named the capital city Addis Ababa. Her military strategy and organization were pivotal in Ethiopia successfully resisting colonization.

Thandiwe

Meaning: Beloved
Origin: African
Influential Person: Melanie Thandiwe Newton Parker OBE aka Thandie Newton – Award-winning British actress.

Tiana

Meaning: Follower of Christ
Origin: English
Influential Person: Tiana – The first Black Disney Princess.

Tiffany

Meaning: Manifestation of God
Origin: Greek
Influential Person: Tiffany Haddish – Award-winning actress, comedian, and author.

Tyra

Meaning: God of the battle
Origin: Norse
Influential Person: Tyra Banks – Model, producer, and businesswoman. She was the first Black woman to feature on the covers of GQ and the Sports Illustrated Swimsuit Issue.

U

Ursula

Meaning: Bear
Origin: Latin
Influential Person: Ursula Burns – First Black woman to become CEO of a Fortune 500 company.

V

Vanessa

Meaning: Butterfly
Origin: Greek
Influential Person: Vanessa Williams – Award-winning singer and actress.

Venus

Meaning: Roman Goddess Of Love. Also a planet in our solar system (2nd closest to the sun)
Origin: Greek
Influential Person: Venus Williams – Highly decorated tennis player.

Viola

Meaning: Derived from Violet meaning purple
Origin: Latin
Influential Person: Viola Davis – Award-winning actress and the youngest and first Black person to receive the "Triple Crown of Acting" (an Academy Award, an Emmy Award, and a Tony award (of which she has won 2)).

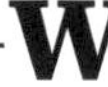

W

Wendy

Meaning: Friend
Origin: English
Influential Person: Wendy Williams – American broadcaster, TV personality, and entrepreneur.

Whitney

Meaning: White island
Origin: English
Influential Person: Whitney Houston – Grammy award-winning artist. She was one of the best-selling (200m+ records worldwide) and most awarded artists of all time.

Whoopi

Meaning: Celebration
Origin: English
Influential Person: Whoopi Goldberg – Award-winning actress and TV personality. She is one of 16 people to have won the "Grand Slam" of show business (A Tony Award, an Emmy award, a Grammy, and an Academy Award).

Willow

Meaning: Slender, graceful
Origin: English
Influential Person: Willow Smith – Award-winning artist and daughter of Will Smith and Jada Pinkett-Smith.

Wilma

Meaning: Resolute protection
Origin: Germanic
Influential Person: Wilma Rudolph – The fastest woman in the world (in her day) and the first American woman to win 3 Olympic gold medals.

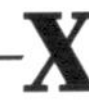

Xiomara

Meaning: Famous in battle
Origin: Spanish
Influential Person: Xiomara Fortuna – Dominican singer & composer.

Y

Yevette/Yvette

Meaning: Yew tree
Origin: German, French
Influential Person: Yvette Marie aka Chaka Khan – Grammy award-winning American singer and songwriter and the "Queen of Funk".

Z

Zadie

Meaning: Prosperous, fortunate
Origin: Arabic
Influential Person: Zadie Smith – Best-selling and award-winning British author.

Zendaya

Meaning: Be thankful
Origin: African – Bantu of Zimbabwe
Influential Person: Zendaya Maree Stoermer Coleman – Emmy award-winning actress & singer.

Zora

Meaning: Dawn
Origin: Arabic
Influential Person: Zora Neale Hurston – American author. Her book "Their Eyes Were Watching God" is considered a classic of the Harlem Renaissance.

Zuri

Meaning: Beautiful
Origin: African
Influential Person: Zuri Tibby – American Model and the first Black model to be a spokesperson for Victoria Secret's PINK.

POPULAR

"Remember that a person's name is to that person the sweetest and most important sound in any language."

Girl ♀

A

Aaliyah
Meaning: Sublime, exalted, noble, rising
Origin: Arabic

Adeline
Meaning: Noble
Origin: French

Adeola
Meaning: The crown brings honor
Origin: African - Nigeria

Africa
Meaning: From Africa
Origin: African

Akari
Meaning: Light
Origin: Japanese

Akinyi
Meaning: One who was born in morning
Origin: Unknown

Akio
Meaning: Bright, clear
Origin: Japanese

Alaina
Meaning: Precious
Origin: Hawaiian

Alexandra
Meaning: Defender of men
Origin: Greek

Alexis
Meaning: Helper, defender
Origin: Greek

Aliyah
Meaning: Ascending, exalted, elevated
Origin: Arabic

Ama
Meaning: Born on Saturday
Origin: African - Ghana

Amaris
Meaning: Promised by God
Origin: Hebrew

Amber
Meaning: Jewel
Origin: Arabic

Ambrose
Meaning: Immortal
Origin: Latin

Angel
Meaning: Messenger
Origin: Greek

Arianna
Meaning: Most holy
Origin: Latin

Ariel
Meaning: Lion of God
Origin: Hebrew

Asher
Meaning: Happy, blessed
Origin: Hebrew

Ashley
Meaning: The Greek Goddess of wild animals
Origin: Greek

Asia
Meaning: Sunrise
Origin: Hebrew

Ava
Meaning: Bird
Origin: Latin

Avayah
Meaning: One who has arrived
Origin: Sanskrit

B

Bali
Meaning: Strength
Origin: Indonesia

Bella
Meaning: Beautiful
Origin: Latin

Beyoncé
Meaning: Beyond others
Origin: Creole

Blair
Meaning: Field, plain
Origin: Scottish

Blaire
Meaning: Field of battle
Origin: Scottish

Bree
Meaning: Noble, power
Origin: Irish

C

Cairo
Meaning: Victorious
Origin: Arabic

Caliana
Meaning: A Moorish princess
Origin: Arabic

Carey
Meaning: From the fort
Origin: irish

Carina
Meaning: Dear one
Origin: Spanish

Casey
Meaning: Vigilant
Origin: Gaelic

Chakra
Meaning: Energy center of the body
Origin: Arabic

Chantelle
Meaning: Singer, to sing
Origin: French

Charity
Meaning: Caring, kindness
Origin: Latin

Charlotte
Meaning: Free
Origin: French

Cheyenne
Meaning: Unintelligible speaker
Origin: Native American

China
Meaning: Qin's kingdom
Origin: China

Chloe
Meaning: Blooming
Origin: Greek

Ciara
Meaning: Dark haired
Origin: Irish

Clara
Meaning: Brilliant, bright
Origin: Latin

Courtney
Meaning: From the court
Origin: English

D

Dayo
Meaning: Happiness has come
Origin: African

Delta
Meaning: Born fourth
Origin: Greek

Demi
Meaning: Half
Origin: French

Denelle
Meaning: God is my judge
Origin: American

Deon
Meaning: God
Origin: Greek

Desiree
Meaning: Much desired
Origin: French

Destiny
Meaning: Fate
Origin: English

Dionne
Meaning: Divine
Origin: Greek

Dominica
Meaning: Belonging to the Lord
Origin: Latin

E

Ebony
Meaning: Black wood
Origin: English

Elana
Meaning: Shining light, tree
Origin: Greek

Elara
Meaning: One of the moons of Jupiter
Origin: Greek

Elektra
Meaning: Shining
Origin: Greek

Ella
Meaning: Goddess
Origin: Hebrew

Elon
Meaning: Oak tree
Origin: Hebrew

Eshe
Meaning: Life
Origin: African

Etta
Meaning: Keeper of the hearth
Origin: French

Eva
Meaning: Life
Origin: Hebrew

F

Faith
Meaning: Complete trust, devotion
Origin: English

Fara
Meaning: Lovely, pleasant
Origin: Arabic

Felicia
Meaning: Fortunate, happy
Origin: Latin

G

Gabriela
Meaning: God is my strength
Origin: Hebrew

Gemma
Meaning: Precious stone
Origin: Italian

Genesis
Meaning: The beginning
Origin: Greek

Ghana
Meaning: A country in Africa. The word means "warrior king"
Origin: African

Gianna
Meaning: The Lord is gracious
Origin: Italian

Giselle
Meaning: Pledge
Origin: French

Grace
Meaning: Charm, goodness, generosity
Origin: Latin

H

Halle
Meaning: Ruler, heroine
Origin: Scandinavian

Harmony
Meaning: Unity
Origin: Greek

Honey

Meaning: Sweet
Origin: American

I

Imani

Meaning: Faith
Origin: Swahili

Imogen

Meaning: Innocent
Origin: Latin

India

Meaning: River
Origin: Unknown

Isla

Meaning: Island
Origin: Scottish

Isobel

Meaning: God is oath
Origin: Hebrew

Issa

Meaning: Jesus
Origin: Arabic

Ivy

Meaning: Faithfulness
Origin: English

Ixia

Meaning: South African flower
Origin: African

J

Jada

Meaning: The knowing one, wise
Origin: Hebrew

Jade

Meaning: Stone of the side
Origin: Spanish

Jaden

Meaning: God has heard
Origin: Hebrew

Jaelynn

Meaning: Supplanter
Origin: American

Jamila

Meaning: Beautiful, elegant
Origin: Arabic

Jana

Meaning: God is gracious
Origin: Hebrew

Jasmine
Meaning: Gift from God
Origin: Persian

Jennifer
Meaning: Fair one
Origin: Cornish

Joe
Meaning: God will give
Origin: Hebrew

Jordan
Meaning: Flowing down
Origin: Hebrew

Jordyn
Meaning: To flow down
Origin: Hebrew

K

Kali
Meaning: Black
Origin: Sanskrit

Kamala
Meaning: Lotus flower
Origin: Indian

Kara
Meaning: Beloved
Origin: Italian

Karasi
Meaning: Full of life and wisdom
Origin: African

Kayla
Meaning: Crown
Origin: Arabic

Kelis
Meaning: Beautiful
Origin: American

Kenya
Meaning: Country in Africa
Origin: Africa

Keshon
Meaning: God is merciful
Origin: English

Kezia
Meaning: Cassia tree
Origin: Hebrew

Kiana
Meaning: Divine
Origin: Hawaiian

Kya
Meaning: Diamond in the sky
Origin: African

L

Laila
Meaning: Night, dark
Origin: Arabic

Latasha
Meaning: Born on Christmas Day
Origin: American

Lateisha
Meaning: Joyful, happy
Origin: English

Leona
Meaning: Lion
Origin: Latin

Logan
Meaning: Little hollow
Origin: Scottish

Lola
Meaning: Sorrows
Origin: Spanish

Luna
Meaning: Moon
Origin: Latin

Lyla
Meaning: Island beauty
Origin: British

Lyra
Meaning: A small constellation
Origin: Greek

M

Mae
Meaning: After the Roman Goddess of spring growth
Origin: Latin

Maia
Meaning: Great
Origin: Latin

Maisha
Meaning: Alive and well
Origin: Arabic

Maria
Meaning: Star of the sea
Origin: Latin

Marley
Meaning: Lake Meadow
Origin: English

Maya
Meaning: Water
Origin: Hebrew

Meagan
Meaning: Pearl
Origin: Welsh

Meghan
Meaning: Pearl
Origin: Welsh

Melody
Meaning: Song, music
Origin: French

Mercedes
Meaning: Mercies
Origin: Latin

Mia
Meaning: Mine
Origin: Hebrew

Mica
Meaning: Loved friend
Origin: Mexican

Mila
Meaning: Favored
Origin: Spanish

Mina
Meaning: Love
Origin: German

Mishon/Michonne
Meaning: A Kind gift from God
Origin: Hebrew

Misty
Meaning: Covered with mist, dew
Origin: English

Monique
Meaning: Advisor
Origin: French

Montana
Meaning: Mountain
Origin: Unknown

N

Nailah
Meaning: Successful
Origin: Arabic

Naimah
Meaning: Peaceful, comfort, tranquility
Origin: Arabic

Naomi
Meaning: Pleasantness
Origin: Hebrew

Neo/Neyo
Meaning: Gift
Origin: African/American

Neriah
Meaning: Lamp of the Lord
Origin: Hebrew

Nevaeh
Meaning: Heaven (spelt backwards)
Origin: American

Niara
Meaning: Utmost purpose
Origin: African–Swahili

Nikki
Meaning: Victory of the people
Origin: American

Nila
Meaning: Blue
Origin: India

Niobe
Meaning: Fern
Origin: Greek

Noel
Meaning: Born on Christmas
Origin: French

Nora
Meaning: Honor
Origin: Latin

Nya
Meaning: Purpose
Origin: African–Swahili

Nyah
Meaning: Lustrous
Origin: African–Swahili

Nyla
Meaning: Champion
Origin: British

Nylah
Meaning: Cloud
Origin: Gaelic

Nyx
Meaning: Night
Origin: Greek

O

Ocean
Meaning: Sea
Origin: Greek

Octavia
Meaning: Eighth
Origin: Latin

Olivia
Meaning: Olive tree
Origin: Latin

Onika
Meaning: A courageous soldier
Origin: Sanskrit

Oralia
Meaning: Golden
Origin: French

Orianna
Meaning: Sunrise
Origin: Latin

P

Pandora
Meaning: All gifts, talented
Origin: Greek

Phoenix
Meaning: Dark red
Origin: Greek

Psalm
Meaning: Song
Origin: Greek

R

Rayne
Meaning: Song
Origin: Scandinavian

Reina
Meaning: Queen
Origin: Unknown

Remi
Meaning: Oarsman
Origin: French

Renee
Meaning: Reborn
Origin: Unknown

Rhea
Meaning: Flowing stream. Also, one of the moons of Saturn
Origin: Greek

Rihanna
Meaning: Great queen
Origin: Irish

Riley
Meaning: Courageous
Origin: British

Rio
Meaning: River
Origin: Spanish

Rosa
Meaning: Rose
Origin: Spanish

Ruby
Meaning: A deep red precious stone
Origin: Latin

Rumi
Meaning: Beauty
Origin: Japanese

S

Saffron
Meaning: A yellow flower and spice
Origin: Arabic

Saint
Meaning: Holy person
Origin: American

Sakari
Meaning: Sweet
Origin: Native American

Sapphire
Meaning: Blue. Also a jewel and birthstone of September
Origin: Hebrew

Sarai
Meaning: My lady, princess
Origin: Hebrew

Sasha
Meaning: Defending warrior
Origin: Russian

Seanna
Meaning: God is gracious
Origin: Irish

Serena
Meaning: Tranquil
Origin: Latin

Shanice
Meaning: God is merciful
Origin: Hebrew

Shayla
Meaning: From the fairy palace
Origin: Gaelic

Shiloh
Meaning: Tranquil
Origin: Hebrew

Shonda
Meaning: God is gracious
Origin: American

Simone
Meaning: God has heard
Origin: Hebrew

Stormy
Meaning: Impetuous nature
Origin: American

T

Taiga
Meaning: Large, big
Origin: Japanese

Tamah
Meaning: Innocent, honest
Origin: Hebrew

Tamara/Tamera
Meaning: Date
Origin: Hebrew

Taraji
Meaning: Hope
Origin: African

Tayen
Meaning: New moon
Origin: Native American

Tia
Meaning: Princess, goddess
Origin: Greek

Tiana
Meaning: Follower of Christ
Origin: English

True
Meaning: Genuine, loyal
Origin: English

Tyra
Meaning: God of the battle
Origin: Norse

U

Uliana
Meaning: Youthful, soft-haired
Origin: Russian

V

Venus
Meaning: Roman Goddess of love. Also a planet in our solar system (2nd closest to the sun)
Origin: Greek

Viola
Meaning: Derived from Violet meaning purple
Origin: Latin

W

Winter
Meaning: Cold season
Origin: American

X

Xiomara
Meaning: Famous in battle
Origin: Spanish

Xoey
Meaning: Life
Origin: Greek

Y

Yara
Meaning: Small butterfly
Origin: Arabic

Yasmina
Meaning: A beautiful flower that shines
Origin: Arabic

Z

Zahara
Meaning: To shine, flower
Origin: Hebrew

Zahra
Meaning: White, light
Origin: Arabic

Zaira
Meaning: Radiance
Origin: Arabic

Zalika
Meaning: Well born
Origin: African–Swahili

Zari
Meaning: Golden
Origin: Arabic

Zariah
Meaning: Radiance
Origin: Arabic

Zen

Meaning: Meditation
Origin: Japanese

Zendaya

Meaning: Be thankful
Origin: African–Bantu of Zimbabwe

Zora

Meaning: Dawn
Origin: Arabic

Zunaira

Meaning: Guiding light
Origin: Arabic

ARABIC

"And when the heart loves something, the eyes see it as Paradise."

Girl ♀

A

Aaliyah
Meaning: Sublime, exalted, noble, rising
Origin: Arabic

Adila
Meaning: Fair
Origin: Arabic

Afeni
Meaning: Health
Origin: Arabic

Afyia
Meaning: Good health
Origin: Arabic

Aiesha
Meaning: Alive and well
Origin: Arabic

Aisha
Meaning: Alive and well
Origin: Arabic

Akilah
Meaning: Intelligent
Origin: Arabic

Aliyah
Meaning: Ascending, exalted, elevated
Origin: Arabic

Aman
Meaning: Security, peace
Origin: Arabic

Amana
Meaning: Security, peace
Origin: Arabic

Amani
Meaning: Wishes
Origin: Arabic

Amber
Meaning: Jewel
Origin: Arabic

Amel
Meaning: Hope
Origin: Arabic

Amina
Meaning: Honest, faithful
Origin: Arabic

Ara
Meaning: King, brings rain
Origin: Arabic

Arusi
Meaning: Marriage, bride
Origin: Arabic

Ayeesha
Meaning: Alive and well
Origin: Arabic

Azalea
Meaning: Democracy, freedom
Origin: Arabic

B

Bahira
Meaning: Dazzling, brilliant
Origin: Arabic

Bari'ah
Meaning: Excelling
Origin: Arabic

Bashira
Meaning: Joyful
Origin: Arabic

C

Cairo
Meaning: Victorious
Origin: Arabic

Caliana
Meaning: A Moorish princess
Origin: Arabic

Caylie
Meaning: Slim and Fair, beloved
Origin: Arabic

Chakra
Meaning: Energy center of the body
Origin: Arabic

D

Damina
Meaning: Lady
Origin: Arabic

Daneen
Meaning: Princess
Origin: Arabic

E

Eiliyah

Meaning: Beautiful one to grow in peace and love with God
Origin: Arabic

Emna

Meaning: Believing
Origin: Arabic

Ezzah

Meaning: A person who gives the honor
Origin: Arabic

F

Fadilah

Meaning: Virtue, distinguished
Origin: Arabic

Faizah

Meaning: Victorious, successful one
Origin: Arabic

Fara

Meaning: Lovely, pleasant
Origin: Arabic

Fari

Meaning: Pretty, beautiful
Origin: Arabic

Faridah

Meaning: Exceptional, unique
Origin: Arabic

G

Gamila

Meaning: Beautiful
Origin: Arabic

Ghadah

Meaning: Beautiful
Origin: Arabic

Ghayda

Meaning: Young and delicate
Origin: Arabic

H

Habibah
Meaning: Beloved
Origin: Arabic

Hadia
Meaning: Leader, guide
Origin: Arabic

Hadiyyah
Meaning: Gift
Origin: Arabic

Halima
Meaning: Patient
Origin: Arabic

Hania
Meaning: Happy
Origin: Arabic

Hasana
Meaning: Beautiful
Origin: Arabic

I

Ifrah
Meaning: To make a person happy
Origin: Arabic

Inaya
Meaning: God Answered
Origin: Hebrew

Issa
Meaning: Jesus
Origin: Arabic

J

Jala
Meaning: Shining, bringing to light
Origin: Arabic

Jamila
Meaning: Beautiful, elegant
Origin: Arabic

Jemila
Meaning: Beautiful
Origin: Arabic

Jumanah
Meaning: Pearl
Origin: Arabic

K

Kabira
Meaning: Noble, great
Origin: Arabic

Kadija
Meaning: Early baby, trustworthy
Origin: Arabic

Kadisha
Meaning: Early baby
Origin: Arabic

Kalila
Meaning: Beloved
Origin: Arabic

Kamilah
Meaning: Perfect
Origin: Arabic

Karimah
Meaning: Generous
Origin: Arabic

Kayla
Meaning: Crown
Origin: Arabic

Khadijah
Meaning: Premature child
Origin: Arabic

Khalidah
Meaning: Immortal
Origin: Arabic

Khalilah
Meaning: Friend
Origin: Arabic

L

Laila
Meaning: Night, dark
Origin: Arabic

Lama
Meaning: Lips that are dark like the color of the sunset
Origin: Arabic

Lamia
Meaning: Radiant
Origin: Arabic

Lamis
Meaning: Soft, tender woman
Origin: Arabic

Lamya
Meaning: Beautiful dark lips
Origin: Arabic

Latifah
Meaning: Kind, gentle
Origin: Arabic

Layla
Meaning: Night
Origin: Arabic

Leela
Meaning: Night beauty
Origin: Arabic

Leila
Meaning: Night
Origin: Arabic

Lulu
Meaning: Pearl
Origin: Arabic

M

Madihah
Meaning: Praiseworthy
Origin: Arabic

Maha
Meaning: Beautiful eyes
Origin: Arabic

Maisha
Meaning: Alive and well
Origin: Arabic

Malika
Meaning: Queen
Origin: Arabic

Manal
Meaning: Attainment
Origin: Arabic

Maram
Meaning: Desire, wish
Origin: Arabic

Marihah
Meaning: Exceedingly happy, joyful, cheerful
Origin: Arabic

Maysa
Meaning: Graceful
Origin: Arabic

Messina
Meaning: Middle child
Origin: Arabic

Monica
Meaning: Advisor
Origin: Latin

Mukai
Meaning: Most beautiful
Origin: Arabic

Muna
Meaning: Desires, wishes
Origin: Arabic

N

Naeemah

Meaning: Happiness, comfort
Origin: Arabic

Nailah

Meaning: Successful
Origin: Arabic

Naimah

Meaning: Peaceful, comfort, tranquility
Origin: Arabic

Nakia

Meaning: Pure
Origin: Arabic

Nama

Meaning: Gift, present, grace
Origin: Arabic

Niesha

Meaning: Derived from Aisha meaning full of life
Origin: Arabic

O

Oadira

Meaning: Powerful, potent
Origin: Arabic

Orzala

Meaning: Brightness of fire
Origin: Arabic

Oza

Meaning: Strength
Origin: Arabic

P

Parey

Meaning: Face of an angel
Origin: Arabic

Piraya

Meaning: Jewels
Origin: Arabic

Q

Qabila
Meaning: Able, wise
Origin: Arabic

Qadira
Meaning: Powerful, able
Origin: Arabic

Qaifa
Meaning: Sight-reader
Origin: Arabic

Qamara
Meaning: The Moon
Origin: Arabic

R

Radhiya
Meaning: Content
Origin: Arabic

Rashida
Meaning: Rightly guided
Origin: Arabic

Raya
Meaning: Friend to all
Origin: Arabic

Raziya
Meaning: Agreeable
Origin: Arabic

Rukiya
Meaning: She rises high
Origin: Arabic

S

Safa
Meaning: Innocent
Origin: Arabic

Saffron
Meaning: A yellow flower and spice
Origin: Arabic

Safiya/Saffiyyah
Meaning: Pure
Origin: Arabic

Sagirah
Meaning: Little one
Origin: Arabic

Sahara
Meaning: Desert
Origin: Arabic

Saidah
Meaning: Fortunate
Origin: Arabic

Sakina
Meaning: Tranquility
Origin: Arabic

Salama
Meaning: Peace
Origin: Arabic

Salma
Meaning: Peaceful
Origin: Arabic

Samira
Meaning: She who is of pleasant company and loved
Origin: Arabic

Sanai
Meaning: Praise
Origin: Arabic

Satira
Meaning: Modest
Origin: Arabic

Selma
Meaning: Peaceful
Origin: Arabic

Shakia
Meaning: Good-looking
Origin: Arabic

Shakila
Meaning: Beautiful
Origin: Arabic

Shaqueela
Meaning: Beautiful
Origin: Arabic

Sharifa
Meaning: Noble
Origin: Arabic

Shereen
Meaning: Sweet, pleasant
Origin: Arabic

Suhailah
Meaning: Gentle
Origin: Arabic

T

Tahirah
Meaning: Pure
Origin: Arabic

Talayah
Meaning: Golden ray of sun
Origin: Arabic

Tazara
Meaning: One who is elegant
Origin: Arabic

Thuraia
Meaning: Star
Origin: Arabic

Tyesha
Meaning: Alive and well
Origin: Arabic

U

Ulema
Meaning: Intelligent one
Origin: Arabic

Ulyaa
Meaning: High, eminent
Origin: Arabic

Uzma
Meaning: Greatest
Origin: Arabic

V

Vajiha
Meaning: Beautiful woman
Origin: Arabic

Vakila
Meaning: Truth
Origin: Arabic

Valiqa
Meaning: Trustworthy
Origin: Arabic

W

Wafia
Meaning: Rights to full pay
Origin: Arabic

Wajia
Meaning: Melody
Origin: Arabic

Wasiqa
Meaning: Stable, firm
Origin: Arabic

Wazna
Meaning: Petite, intelligent
Origin: Arabic

X

Xarika
Meaning: Life blessing, princess
Origin: Arabic

Xavia
Meaning: Bright, splendid
Origin: Arabic

Xaviera
Meaning: Bright, splendid
Origin: Arabic

Xavon
Meaning: Beautiful
Origin: Arabic

Xeanee
Meaning: The one that cannot be broken
Origin: Arabic

Y

Yadira
Meaning: Suitable, worthy
Origin: Arabic

Yaminah
Meaning: Proper, blessed
Origin: Arabic

Yara
Meaning: Small butterfly
Origin: Arabic

Yasmina
Meaning: A beautiful flower that shines
Origin: Arabic

Yasmine
Meaning: Flower
Origin: Arabic

Z

Zabia
Meaning: Like deer
Origin: Arabic

Zadie
Meaning: Prosperous, fortunate
Origin: Arabic

Zahira
Meaning: Bright, illuminating
Origin: Arabic

Zahra
Meaning: White, light
Origin: Arabic

Zahwa
Meaning: Joy, beauty, happiness
Origin: Arabic

Zaila
Meaning: Power
Origin: Arabic

Zaira
Meaning: Radiance
Origin: Arabic

Zakiyah
Meaning: Pure
Origin: Arabic

Zara
Meaning: Radiance
Origin: Arabic

Zareen
Meaning: Full of expression and smile
Origin: Arabic

Zarene
Meaning: Golden one
Origin: Arabic

Zari
Meaning: Golden
Origin: Arabic

Zarina
Meaning: Golden
Origin: Arabic

Ziya
Meaning: Splendor, glow
Origin: Arabic

Zora
Meaning: Dawn
Origin: Arabic

Zorana

Meaning: Derived from Zora meaning Dawn
Origin: Arabic

Zunaira

Meaning: Guiding light
Origin: Arabic

AFRICAN AMERICAN

"Children are the reward of life." –African Proverb

Girl ♀

A

Afyia

Meaning: Good health
Origin: Arabic

B

Brandy

Meaning: Warm and comforting
Origin: American

Breana, Brianna

Meaning: Noble, high
Origin: Irish

Briona

Meaning: Woman with many virtues
Origin: American

C

Camisha

Meaning: Combination of Camilla meaning religious helper and Alisha meaning noble, kind
Origin: American

Chara

Meaning: Joy, happiness
Origin: Greek

Charmaine

Meaning: Freeman, strong
Origin: English

D

Darnesha
Meaning: Hidden
Origin: Old English

Dashawna
Meaning: God is gracious
Origin: African American

De-Andra
Meaning: Defender of mankind, divine
Origin: African American

Deandra
Meaning: Divine, protector of man
Origin: English

Denelle
Meaning: God is my judge
Origin: American

Denisha
Meaning: Follower of Dionysius
Origin: French

Dericia
Meaning: Athletic
Origin: American

E

Elayah
Meaning: Gifted with prosperity
Origin: African American

F

Fantasia
Meaning: Vivid imagination
Origin: Italian

G

Gaynelle
Meaning: Happy
Origin: American

I

Issa
Meaning: Jesus
Origin: Arabic

J

Ja-Lisa
Meaning: God's promise
Origin: American

Jaamise
Meaning: Beautiful girl
Origin: African American

Jaelynn
Meaning: Supplanter
Origin: American

Jamaa
Meaning: Supplanter
Origin: Hebrew

Janaya
Meaning: God has answered
Origin: English

Janelle
Meaning: God is merciful
Origin: Hebrew

K

Kalisa
Meaning: One who has given herself to God
Origin: American

Keandra
Meaning: Variation of Kendra meaning knowledge
Origin: Old English

Keisha
Meaning: Her life, woman
Origin: American

Keysha
Meaning: Her life, woman
Origin: American

Kiona/Kionia
Meaning: Brown hills
Origin: American

L

Lacrecia/Lacricia
Meaning: Succeed
Origin: Latin

Ladonna
Meaning: Lady
Origin: American

Lakeisha
Meaning: Favorite
Origin: American

Lamesha
Meaning: Queen
Origin: African American

Lanelle
Meaning: Precious
Origin: American

Laqueta
Meaning: The quiet one
Origin: African American

Laquinda
Meaning: Light, deity
Origin: Spanish

Laquisha
Meaning: Joyful, happy
Origin: English

Lasean
Meaning: God is gracious
Origin: American

Lashawna
Meaning: God's grace
Origin: American

Lashonda
Meaning: God is gracious
Origin: American

Latasha
Meaning: Born on Christmas Day
Origin: American

Latoyah
Meaning: Victory
Origin: Unknown

M

Madea
Meaning: Matriarch of the family
Origin: African

Maliyah
Meaning: Beloved
Origin: Hawaiian

Mekelle
Meaning: Who is like God?
Origin: African American

Mikeya
Meaning: Who is like God?
Origin: African American

N

Nakai
Meaning: One who wanders
Origin: Native American

Nakeisha
Meaning: Her life
Origin: African American

Natoya
Meaning: One who can dance
Origin: American/African

Necie
Meaning: Passionate, intense, fiery
Origin: Jamaican

Neo/Neyo
Meaning: Gift
Origin: African/American

Nevaeh
Meaning: Heaven (spelled backward)
Origin: American

Nia
Meaning: Purpose, goal
Origin: African–Swahili

Niara
Meaning: Utmost purpose
Origin: African–Swahili

Niesha
Meaning: Derived from Aisha meaning full of life
Origin: Arabic

Nikeisha
Meaning: Derived from Keisha meaning great joy
Origin: American

Nikki
Meaning: Victory of the people
Origin: American

Nyesha
Meaning: Pure
Origin: American

O

Ophrah
Meaning: Fawn
Origin: Hebrew

P

Phoenicia
Meaning: Red, purple
Origin: Israel

Q

Quanesia
Meaning: Life
Origin: Jamaican/ African American

Quansha
Meaning: Life
Origin: Jamaican

Queisha
Meaning: Spice Tree
Origin: African

Quisha
Meaning: Having a beautiful mind
Origin: American

R

Raimy
Meaning: Celebration
Origin: American

Rakesha
Meaning: To guard, the Moon
Origin: American/Indian

Ranielle
Meaning: God is my judge
Origin: American/African

Rashawn
Meaning: God is gracious
Origin: Hebrew

Rashona
Meaning: God's favorite
Origin: American

Rayhelle
Meaning: Goodwill
Origin: African American

Reshay
Meaning: A gift
Origin: Jamaican

Ricki
Meaning: Brave ruler
Origin: American

Rochelle
Meaning: Little Rock, rest
Origin: German

Ronna
Meaning: Bringing victory
Origin: American

S

Shalonda
Meaning: Derived from Yolanda meaning violet
Origin: African American

Shamica/Shamika
Meaning: Majestic
Origin: American

Shandee
Meaning: Goddess
Origin: American

Shaneta
Meaning: Gracious
Origin: American

Shaniqua
Meaning: Gift of God
Origin: African American

Shanique
Meaning: God is gracious
Origin: American

Shantewa
Meaning: God's present
Origin: African

Shaquana
Meaning: Truth in life
Origin: African American

Shardea
Meaning: Honor earns the crown
Origin: African

Sharonda
Meaning: A fertile plain
Origin: Hebrew

Shauna
Meaning: God is gracious
Origin: Irish

Shaundra
Meaning: Stones
Origin: American

Shenice
Meaning: God is gracious
Origin: African American

Shonda
Meaning: God is gracious
Origin: American

Shontaya
Meaning: God is gracious
Origin: American

Simone
Meaning: God has heard
Origin: Hebrew

T

Taheisha
Meaning: Joy
Origin: American

Takeisha
Meaning: From Keisha meaning great joy
Origin: American

Takira
Meaning: Sun
Origin: American

Taleisha
Meaning: Blooming life
Origin: African American

Tameca
Meaning: Sweet
Origin: American

Tamecia
Meaning: Sweet
Origin: American

Tanesha/Taneisha
Meaning: Worthy of praise
Origin: African American

Tanginika
Meaning: Lake Goddess
Origin: American

Tashelle
Meaning: Born on Christmas Day
Origin: American

Tashina
Meaning: Beauty of the mountains
Origin: American

Teona
Meaning: Princess
Origin: Jamaican

Tinashe
Meaning: God is with us
Origin: African

Tonya
Meaning: Praiseworthy
Origin: Unknown

Trinika
Meaning: Pure
Origin: African American

Tyonna
Meaning: Princess
Origin: American

V

Velda
Meaning: Power, ruler
Origin: American

W

Wakeisha
Meaning: Derived from Keisha meaning great joy
Origin: Jamaican

Y

Yetty
Meaning: Ruler of the household
Origin: African American

Z

Zabrina
Meaning: Fruitful desert flower
Origin: American

Zahira
Meaning: Bright, illuminating
Origin: Arabic

Zekia
Meaning: Pure
Origin: Jamaican

MODERN

"Words have meanings. Names have power."

Girl ♀

A

Ada
Meaning: Noble, happy
Origin: German

Adira
Meaning: Strong, powerful
Origin: Hebrew

Adjoa
Meaning: Belonging to the sun
Origin: India

Afyia
Meaning: Good health
Origin: Arabic

Ahanti
Meaning: Eternal, indestructible, warlike
Origin: Hindi

Aina
Meaning: Love, affection, love of greens
Origin: Japanese

Aiyana
Meaning: Eternal flower, blossom
Origin: Native American

Akari
Meaning: Light
Origin: Japanese

Akina
Meaning: Spring flower
Origin: Japanese

Alaia
Meaning: Sublime
Origin: Arabic

Alaska
Meaning: Great land
Origin: American

Aleshanee
Meaning: She plays all the time
Origin: Native American

Alessia
Meaning: Defending warrior
Origin: Italian

Alexa
Meaning: Defender of mankind
Origin: Greek

Alexandra
Meaning: Defender of men
Origin: Greek

Alexandria
Meaning: Defender of mankind
Origin: Unknown

Alexis
Meaning: Helper, defender
Origin: Greek

Alicia
Meaning: Noble, kind
Origin: Old German

Alina
Meaning: Light
Origin: Russian

Alisa
Meaning: Great happiness
Origin: Hebrew

Alisha
Meaning: Noble, kind
Origin: Sanskrit

Alora
Meaning: My dream
Origin: African

Alyssa
Meaning: Noble
Origin: English

Amahle
Meaning: The beautiful one
Origin: African - South Africa

Amaka
Meaning: Noble, kind
Origin: English

Amanda
Meaning: Lovable
Origin: Greek

Amarantha
Meaning: Unfading
Origin: Greek

Amaryllis
Meaning: Sparkle
Origin: Latin

Amaya
Meaning: Night rain
Origin: Japanese

Amelia
Meaning: Immortal
Origin: Greek

Ameyalli
Meaning: Fountain
Origin: Native American

Anastasia
Meaning: Resurrection, revival
Origin: Greek

Annika
Meaning: Grace
Origin: Hebrew

Anya
Meaning: Favored, grace
Origin: Russian

Aoko
Meaning: Blue child
Origin: Japanese

April
Meaning: To open
Origin: Latin

Aquene
Meaning: Peace
Origin: Native American

Ara
Meaning: King, brings rain
Origin: Arabic

Arali
Meaning: The base of the Earth
Origin: Greek

Ari
Meaning: Lion
Origin: Scandinavian

Arielle
Meaning: Lion of God
Origin: Hebrew

Armani
Meaning: Warrior
Origin: Italian

Artemis
Meaning: Butcher, after the Greek Goddess of the hunt
Origin: Greek

Athena
Meaning: After the Greek Goddess of war & wisdom
Origin: Greek

Audi
Meaning: Last daughter
Origin: African

Aurelia
Meaning: Golden
Origin: Latin

Auri
Meaning: Golden
Origin: Latin

Aurora
Meaning: Dawn
Origin: Latin

Avayah
Meaning: One who has arrived
Origin: Sanskrit

Avery
Meaning: Ruler of the elves, wise
Origin: French

Ayla
Meaning: Deer
Origin: Hebrew

Azana
Meaning: Ultimate
Origin: African

B

Bailey
Meaning: Agent of the law
Origin: Old English

Bambi
Meaning: Child
Origin: Italian

Beau
Meaning: Beautiful
Origin: French

Belicia
Meaning: God is my oath
Origin: Spanish

Benecia
Meaning: Blessed one
Origin: Spanish

Benita
Meaning: Blessed
Origin: Italian

Blaire
Meaning: Field of battle
Origin: Scottish

Blossom
Meaning: Flower like
Origin: English

Boston
Meaning: By the woods
Origin: Unknown

Breana/Brianna
Meaning: Noble, high
Origin: Irish

Bree
Meaning: Noble, power
Origin: Irish

Breona
Meaning: Strong, virtuous, noble
Origin: English

Bridgitte
Meaning: Exalted one
Origin: Gaelic

Brielle
Meaning: God is my strength
Origin: French

Briona
Meaning: A woman with many virtues
Origin: American

Bron
Meaning: Brown, dark
Origin: French

Brooke
Meaning: Brook, stream
Origin: English

Brooklyn
Meaning: Beautiful brook
Origin: Unknown

Bryony
Meaning: To sprout
Origin: Latin

Butterfly
Meaning: After a butterfly
Origin: Old English

C

Cacey
Meaning: Vigilant
Origin: Irish

Cadena
Meaning: With rhythm
Origin: English

Calandra
Meaning: Singing bird
Origin: Greek

Caliana
Meaning: A Moorish princess
Origin: Arabic

Camilla
Meaning: Religious helper
Origin: French

Camille
Meaning: Religious helper
Origin: French

Caprice
Meaning: Playful, whimsical
Origin: Italian

Cardia
Meaning: Heart
Origin: Greek

Carey
Meaning: From the fort
Origin: irish

Cari
Meaning: Beloved
Origin: Welsh

Caryne
Meaning: Pure
Origin: English

Cassandra
Meaning: Shining, excelling
Origin: Greek

Cassia
Meaning: Cinnamon
Origin: Greek

Catalina
Meaning: Pure
Origin: Spanish

Catori
Meaning: Spirit
Origin: Native American

Caylie
Meaning: Slim and fair, beloved
Origin: Arabic

Cecilia
Meaning: Blind
Origin: Latin

Chandelle
Meaning: Candle
Origin: French

Chase
Meaning: Huntsman
Origin: French

Chelsea
Meaning: Chalk landing place
Origin: Unknown

Cherry
Meaning: Cherry fruit
Origin: British

Chiara
Meaning: Bright, luminous
Origin: Italian

Chicago
Meaning: Onion
Origin: Unknown

Chloe
Meaning: Blooming
Origin: Greek

Cinnamon
Meaning: A spice
Origin: Greek

Cleona
Meaning: Father's glory
Origin: Greek

Condoleeza
Meaning: With sweetness
Origin: Italian

Coraline
Meaning: Coral of the sea
Origin: American

Cori
Meaning: Maiden
Origin: Greek

Corine
Meaning: Maiden
Origin: English

Cosmo
Meaning: Harmony, order
Origin: Italian

Cyrah
Meaning: Throne
Origin: Persian

Cyran
Meaning: Spear
Origin: Latin

D

Dakota
Meaning: Allies, friends
Origin: Native American

Dallas
Meaning: The meadow dwelling
Origin: Unknown

Darcy
Meaning: Dark haired
Origin: Irish

Deana
Meaning: From the valley
Origin: English

Deandra
Meaning: Divine, protector of man
Origin: English

Deja
Meaning: Already
Origin: Spanish

Delphine
Meaning: From the place called Delphi
Origin: Green

Demi
Meaning: Half
Origin: French

Denelle
Meaning: God is my judge
Origin: American

Denisha
Meaning: Follower of Dionysius
Origin: French

Deriçia
Meaning: Athletic
Origin: American

Desirae
Meaning: Much desired
Origin: French

Desiree
Meaning: Much desired
Origin: French

Devon
Meaning: From Devonshire
Origin: English

Diamond
Meaning: High value, brilliant
Origin: English

Dion
Meaning: Divine
Origin: Greek

Dione
Meaning: Divine queen
Origin: Greek

Dior
Meaning: Golden
Origin: French

Divine
Meaning: Heavenly
Origin: Latin

Dominica
Meaning: Belonging to the Lord
Origin: Latin

Dorene
Meaning: Gift
Origin: Greek

Drina
Meaning: Defender of mankind
Origin: Spanish

Dune
Meaning: Brown skinned soldier
Origin: Scottish

Dyani
Meaning: Deer
Origin: Native American

Dyanna
Meaning: Divine
Origin: Latin

E

Eba
Meaning: Life
Origin: Hebrew

Eden
Meaning: Place of pleasure
Origin: Hebrew

Edith
Meaning: Prosperous in war
Origin: English

Elayah
Meaning: Gifted with prosperity
Origin: African American

Eleasha
Meaning: God is salvation
Origin: Hebrew

Elektra
Meaning: Shining
Origin: Greek

Eliana
Meaning: God has answered
Origin: Hebrew

Elianna
Meaning: God has answered
Origin: Hebrew

Elissia
Meaning: God is my salvation
Origin: Hebrew

Ella
Meaning: Goddess
Origin: Hebrew

Elle
Meaning: She
Origin: French

Elois
Meaning: Famous warrior
Origin: German

Eloise
Meaning: Famous warrior
Origin: German

Elvan
Meaning: Colorful
Origin: Turkish

Enola
Meaning: Magnolia
Origin: Native American

Erica
Meaning: Eternal ruler
Origin: Norse

Evangelia
Meaning: Bringer of good news
Origin: Greek

Evelyn
Meaning: Desired
Origin: English

Evette
Meaning: Living one
Origin: Hebrew

Evie
Meaning: Life
Origin: Hebrew

Evy
Meaning: Life, breathe
Origin: Hebrew

F

Fantasia
Meaning: Vivid imagination
Origin: Italian

Faye
Meaning: Fairy
Origin: English

Felicia
Meaning: Fortunate, happy
Origin: Latin

Fen
Meaning: Perfume
Origin: Chinese

Fifi
Meaning: Jehovah increases
Origin: French

Finesse
Meaning: One who is smooth
Origin: American

Fleur
Meaning: Flower
Origin: French

Florence
Meaning: Blossoming, flourishing
Origin: Latin

Florentina
Meaning: Blooming, flowering
Origin: Latin

Floressa
Meaning: Flower
Origin: Latin

Floretta
Meaning: Flower
Origin: Latin

Franchesca
Meaning: Free
Origin: Italian

G

Gabrielle
Meaning: God is my strength
Origin: Hebrew

Gaia
Meaning: Mother Earth
Origin: Greek

Gaynelle
Meaning: Happy
Origin: American

Gene
Meaning: Born lucky
Origin: Greek

Geneva
Meaning: Juniper berry
Origin: Germanic

Georgia
Meaning: A girl who works the soil
Origin: Greek

Germaine
Meaning: Brother
Origin: French

Ghana
Meaning: A country in Africa. The word means "warrior king"
Origin: African

Ghayda
Meaning: Young and delicate
Origin: Arabic

Gianna
Meaning: The Lord is gracious
Origin: Italian

Ginger
Meaning: Liveliness
Origin: British

Giselle
Meaning: Pledge
Origin: French

Greta
Meaning: Pearl
Origin: German

H

Halima
Meaning: Patient
Origin: Arabic

Halona
Meaning: Happy fortune
Origin: Native American

Hanita
Meaning: Divine grace
Origin: India

Harlow
Meaning: Rock hill
Origin: English

Harper
Meaning: Harp player
Origin: English

Hayden
Meaning: Hay valley
Origin: English

Honey
Meaning: Sweet
Origin: American

I

Ida
Meaning: Industrious one
Origin: German

Inaya
Meaning: God Answered
Origin: Hebrew

Indigo
Meaning: Indian dye
Origin: Greek

Isadora
Meaning: Gift of Isis
Origin: Greek

Israel
Meaning: May God prevail
Origin: Unknown

Ivy
Meaning: Faithfulness
Origin: English

J

Ja-Lisa
Meaning: God's promise
Origin: American

Jacinta
Meaning: Beautiful
Origin: Greek

Jada
Meaning: The knowing one, wise
Origin: Hebrew

Jaelynn
Meaning: Supplanter
Origin: American

Jalen
Meaning: Tranquil
Origin: American

Jalissa
Meaning: Noble natured
Origin: English

Jamila
Meaning: Beautiful, elegant
Origin: Arabic

Janeka
Meaning: God is gracious
Origin: English

Janelle
Meaning: God is merciful
Origin: Hebrew

Janus
Meaning: Gateway
Origin: Latin

Jariah
Meaning: Tributary Lord
Origin: Hebrew

Jaric/Jarrick
Meaning: Strong, fierce
Origin: Jamaican

Jasmine
Meaning: Gift from God
Origin: Persian

Jay
Meaning: Blue crested bird
Origin: Latin

Jaya
Meaning: Victorious
Origin: Indian

Jayla
Meaning: God will protect
Origin: Hebrew

Jazz
Meaning: Derived from Jasmine meaning gift from God
Origin: Persian

Jemma
Meaning: Precious Stone, gem
Origin: English

Jennifer
Meaning: Fair one
Origin: Cornish

Jenue
Meaning: From Jenue in Nigeria
Origin: African

Jessamine
Meaning: Jasmine flower
Origin: Persian/French

Jet
Meaning: Black stone
Origin: British

Jetta
Meaning: Ruler of the house
Origin: Danish

Jewel
Meaning: Delight
Origin: French

Jojo
Meaning: God raises
Origin: Hebrew

Joya
Meaning: Joy
Origin: Latin

Judge
Meaning: Decision maker
Origin: English

Jules
Meaning: Youthful
Origin: French

K

Kacondra
Meaning: One who is bold
Origin: American

Kadija
Meaning: Early baby, trustworthy
Origin: Arabic

Kadisha
Meaning: Early baby
Origin: Arabic

Kaja
Meaning: Pure, echo
Origin: Greek/Estonian

Kalila
Meaning: Beloved
Origin: Arabic

Kalina
Meaning: Flower
Origin: Slavic

Kalisha
Meaning: Fortunate woman
Origin: Latin

Kamala
Meaning: Lotus flower
Origin: Indian

Kamilah
Meaning: Perfect
Origin: Arabic

Kanika
Meaning: An atom, molecule
Origin: Indian

Karah
Meaning: Beloved
Origin: Latin

Karimah
Meaning: Generous
Origin: Arabic

Karla
Meaning: Freewoman
Origin: German

Karma
Meaning: Fate, destiny
Origin: Sanskrit

Kasa
Meaning: Dressed in furs
Origin: Native American

Kasi
Meaning: Shining
Origin: Indian

Kasmira
Meaning: Famous destroyer of peace
Origin: Slavic

Kassiani
Meaning: Cinnamon
Origin: Greek

Kaula
Meaning: Prophet
Origin: Polynesian

Kaya
Meaning: Rock
Origin: Turkish

Kaylen
Meaning: Keeper of the keys
Origin: English

Keandra
Meaning: Variation of Kendra meaning knowledge
Origin: Old English

Keeya
Meaning: Garden flower
Origin: African

Kei
Meaning: Joyful
Origin: Japanese

Keiko
Meaning: Glad, rejoicing child
Origin: Japanese

Kelis
Meaning: Beautiful
Origin: American

Kelsey
Meaning: Victorious ship
Origin: Old English

Kemi
Meaning: To be pampered
Origin: African

Kendal
Meaning: Valley of the river Kent
Origin: English

Kendria
Meaning: Greatest champion
Origin: Welsh

Kenya
Meaning: Country in Africa
Origin: Africa

Keshon
Meaning: God is merciful
Origin: English

Keziah
Meaning: Cassia tree
Origin: Hebrew

Khloe
Meaning: Small green shoot of a plant
Origin: Greek

Kian
Meaning: God is Gracious
Origin: Irish

Kiana
Meaning: Divine
Origin: Hawaiian

Kiara
Meaning: Clear
Origin: Unknown

Kimeya
Meaning: Singing throat
Origin: Native American

Kimi
Meaning: Secret
Origin: Native American

Kingston
Meaning: King's settlement
Origin: British

Kiona/Kionia
Meaning: Brown hills
Origin: American

Kione
Meaning: Someone who comes from nowhere
Origin: African

Kisha
Meaning: Rainfall
Origin: Slavic

Kiyana
Meaning: Deity
Origin: Indian

Kodiak
Meaning: Island
Origin: Russian

Kylie
Meaning: Graceful, beautiful
Origin: Gaelic

Kyra
Meaning: Lord
Origin: Greek

Kyrie
Meaning: Lord
Origin: Greek

Kyrina
Meaning: Lord
Origin: Greek

L

La-juana
Meaning: God is gracious
Origin: American

La-Verne
Meaning: Alder tree grove
Origin: French

Lachelle
Meaning: Who is like God?
Origin: Hebrew

Lacrecia/Lacricia
Meaning: Succeed
Origin: Latin

Ladonna
Meaning: Lady
Origin: American

Laila
Meaning: Night, dark
Origin: Arabic

Lakeisha
Meaning: Favorite
Origin: American

Lakresha
Meaning: Profit
Origin: Jamaican

Lamu
Meaning: Land
Origin: Unknown

Lana
Meaning: Child
Origin: Irish

Laquinda
Meaning: Light, deity
Origin: Spanish

Laquisha
Meaning: Joyful, happy
Origin: English

Lara
Meaning: Protection
Origin: Greek

Larae
Meaning: Grace
Origin: Scottish

Larah
Meaning: Advisor
Origin: English

Larissa
Meaning: Cheerful
Origin: Greek

Lashawna
Meaning: God's grace
Origin: American

Lashonda
Meaning: God is gracious
Origin: American

Lateisha
Meaning: Joyful, happy
Origin: English

Latifah
Meaning: Kind, gentle
Origin: Arabic

Latoria
Meaning: Victorious one
Origin: Spanish

Latorray
Meaning: Victory
Origin: Jamaican

Latoya
Meaning: Victorious one
Origin: Spanish

Latreece
Meaning: Noble
Origin: American/Latin

Latricia
Meaning: Noble
Origin: American/Latin

Lavern
Meaning: Alder tree grove
Origin: French

Lavonne
Meaning: Wood
Origin: English

Leela
Meaning: Night beauty
Origin: Arabic

Legend
Meaning: Story, myth
Origin: English

Leila
Meaning: Night
Origin: Arabic

Leilani
Meaning: Heavenly flower
Origin: Hawaiian

Lenka
Meaning: Torch of light
Origin: Greek

Lennox
Meaning: With many elm trees
Origin: Gaelic

Leonda
Meaning: Lioness
Origin: French

Leonie
Meaning: Lion
Origin: Latin

Lesia
Meaning: Noble
Origin: Latin

Liana
Meaning: To twine around
Origin: French

Liliana
Meaning: Lilly, flower
Origin: Latin

Lily
Meaning: Pure
Origin: Latin

Logan
Meaning: Little hollow
Origin: Scottish

Lomasi
Meaning: Pretty flower
Origin: Native American

London
Meaning: From the great river
Origin: Unknown

Lorraine
Meaning: From the province of Lorraine
Origin: French

Lotus
Meaning: Lotus flower
Origin: Greek

Louella
Meaning: Famous warrior
Origin: German

Louise
Meaning: Famous warrior
Origin: Unknown

Luana
Meaning: Enjoyment
Origin: Hawaiian

Lucinda
Meaning: Light
Origin: Latin

Lucy
Meaning: Light
Origin: Latin

Lumi
Meaning: Snow
Origin: Finnish

Luna
Meaning: Moon
Origin: Latin

Lux
Meaning: Light
Origin: Latin

Luzmina
Meaning: Mine of light
Origin: Spanish

Lynx
Meaning: Brightness
Origin: Greek

Lyra
Meaning: A small constellation
Origin: Greek

M

Madison
Meaning: Gift From God
Origin: English

Magic
Meaning: Full of wonder
Origin: American

Maida
Meaning: Maiden
Origin: English

Manica
Meaning: Jewels
Origin: African

Manuka
Meaning: Tree which produces honey
Origin: Sri Lanka

Marcy
Meaning: Follower of Mars (Roman God of war)
Origin: Latin

Marla
Meaning: Star of the sea
Origin: Latin

Marquita
Meaning: Dedicates to Mars (Roman God of war)
Origin: Latin

Martina
Meaning: Warrior
Origin: Latin

Maxine
Meaning: The greatest
Origin: English/Latin

Maya
Meaning: Water
Origin: Hebrew

Melea
Meaning: Complete, full
Origin: Hebrew

Melody
Meaning: Song, music
Origin: French

Merritt
Meaning: Boundary gate
Origin: English

Meta
Meaning: Pearl
Origin: Greek

Misty
Meaning: Covered with mist, dew
Origin: English

Moana
Meaning: Ocean, sea
Origin: Hawaiian

Montell
Meaning: My ruler
Origin: French

Mya
Meaning: Beloved, great
Origin: Greek

Myla
Meaning: Mild and merciful
Origin: Latin

Myra
Meaning: Myrrh
Origin: Latin/Greek

Mystique
Meaning: Air of mystery
Origin: French

N

Naia
Meaning: Dolphin
Origin: Hawaiian

Nailah
Meaning: Successful
Origin: Arabic

Nairobi
Meaning: Cool water
Origin: Unknown

Nakai
Meaning: One who wanders
Origin: Native American

Nasha
Meaning: Judge
Origin: Persian

Nekesa
Meaning: Born during the harvest
Origin: Unknown

Nella
Meaning: Horn
Origin: Latin

Nevaeh
Meaning: Heaven (spelt backwards)
Origin: American

Nina
Meaning: Favor, grace
Origin: Hebrew

Nisha
Meaning: Night
Origin: Indian

Nishay
Meaning: Night, the night, dark time
Origin: Indian

Nori
Meaning: Belief
Origin: Unknown

Nova
Meaning: New. Also, an astronomical event that causes the sudden appearance of light
Origin: Latin

O

Oceana
Meaning: Ocean
Origin: Greek

Odessa
Meaning: Wrathful
Origin: Greek

Oja
Meaning: Vitality
Origin: Hindi

Onyeka
Meaning: God is the greatest
Origin: African–Nigeria

Ophelia
Meaning: Help
Origin: Greek

Orenda
Meaning: Magic power
Origin: Native American

Orlando
Meaning: Famous throughout the land
Origin: Unknown

P

Palmer
Meaning: Pilgrim
Origin: English

Parisa
Meaning: Like a fairy
Origin: Persian

Persephone
Meaning: Bringer of destruction, to destroy
Origin: Greek

Peyton
Meaning: Fighting-man's estate
Origin: English

Philippa
Meaning: Lover of horses
Origin: Unknown

Precious
Meaning: Of great worth, expensive
Origin: Latin

Prima
Meaning: First
Origin: Latin

Promise
Meaning: A pledge
Origin: English

Prunella
Meaning: Little plum
Origin: Latin

Q

Qamara
Meaning: The Moon
Origin: Arabic

Qianna
Meaning: Gracious
Origin: English

Quanda
Meaning: Queen
Origin: English

Questa
Meaning: One who seeks
Origin: French

Quetzal
Meaning: Large brilliant tail feather
Origin: American

Quinn
Meaning: Descendant of Conn
Origin: Irish

R

Rachel
Meaning: Ewe
Origin: Hebrew

Rachele
Meaning: Ewe, female sheep
Origin: Hebrew

Rada
Meaning: Gladness, joy
Origin: Bulgarian

Rae
Meaning: Ewe
Origin: Hebrew

Raimy
Meaning: Celebration
Origin: American

Rain
Meaning: Rain
Origin: British

Raina
Meaning: Queen
Origin: Latin/Slavic

Rakesha
Meaning: To guard, the Moon
Origin: American/Indian

Ramira
Meaning: Judicious
Origin: Spanish

Ramona
Meaning: Counsel protection
Origin: Spanish/German

Randa
Meaning: Admirable
Origin: English

Raquel
Meaning: Ewe
Origin: Spanish

Raven
Meaning: Dark-haired, wise
Origin: English

Razi
Meaning: Secret
Origin: Hebrew

Reagan
Meaning: Little king
Origin: Irish

Reed
Meaning: Red
Origin: British

Reese
Meaning: Enthusiastic
Origin: Welsh

Reiba
Meaning: To tie
Origin: Unknown

Renell
Meaning: Reborn
Origin: French

Rhonda
Meaning: Noisy
Origin: English

Rhondelle
Meaning: Good lance, spear
Origin: Welsh

River
Meaning: Stream of water that flows to the sea
Origin: English

Roberta
Meaning: Bright fame
Origin: German

Robin
Meaning: Famous, bright
Origin: German

Rochelle
Meaning: Little Rock, rest
Origin: German

Rocket
Meaning: A jet propelled tube
Origin: English

Romy
Meaning: Dew of the sea
Origin: Latin

Ronella
Meaning: Rough island
Origin: Norse

Rosario
Meaning: Rosary
Origin: Spanish

Rose
Meaning: A flower
Origin: Latin

Ruby
Meaning: A deep red precious stone
Origin: Latin

Rukiya
Meaning: She rises high
Origin: Arabic

Rumi
Meaning: Beauty
Origin: Japanese

Ryder
Meaning: Horseman, rider
Origin: English

S

Safari
Meaning: Journey
Origin: African

Saffron
Meaning: A yellow flower and spice
Origin: Arabic

Saint
Meaning: Holy person
Origin: American

Samia
Meaning: Exalted
Origin: Arabic

Santana
Meaning: Follower of St. Ana
Origin: Spanish

Sariah
Meaning: Princess of the Lord
Origin: Unknown

Saturn
Meaning: The Roman God of wealth & agriculture. Also a ringed planet in our solar system
Origin: Latin

Serena
Meaning: Tranquil
Origin: Latin

Shakia
Meaning: Good-looking
Origin: Arabic

Shakila
Meaning: Beautiful
Origin: Arabic

Shareese/Sharise
Meaning: Grace
Origin: Greek

Shea
Meaning: Admirable
Origin: Gaelic

Shenice
Meaning: God is gracious
Origin: African American

Sheree
Meaning: Darling
Origin: French

Shona
Meaning: God is gracious
Origin: Hebrew

Sierra
Meaning: Mountain
Origin: Spanish

Sisi
Meaning: Born on Sunday
Origin: African

Sloan
Meaning: Warrior
Origin: Scottish

Soraya
Meaning: Gem, jewel
Origin: Persian

Stacy
Meaning: Resurrection
Origin: English

Storm
Meaning: Tempest
Origin: British

T

Tahleea
Meaning: Derived from Tahlia meaning Heaven's dew
Origin: Hebrew

Taiga
Meaning: Large, big
Origin: Japanese

Taiwo
Meaning: First twin to taste the world
Origin: African

Taja
Meaning: Crown
Origin: Indian

Talayah
Meaning: Golden ray of sun
Origin: Arabic

Tallulah
Meaning: Leaping water
Origin: Native American

Tasiya
Meaning: Resurrection
Origin: Greek

Tatiana
Meaning: Fairy princess
Origin: Latin

Teana
Meaning: Follower of Christ
Origin: English

Temima
Meaning: Whole
Origin: Hebrew

Thalia
Meaning: Flourishing
Origin: Greek

Tia
Meaning: Princess, Goddess
Origin: Greek

Tiana
Meaning: Follower of Christ
Origin: English

Tiva
Meaning: Dance
Origin: Native American

Tokyo
Meaning: Eastern Capital
Origin: Unknown

Trinity
Meaning: Pertaining to the Holy Trinity of the Father, the Son, and the Holy Spirit
Origin: English

Tyonna
Meaning: Princess
Origin: American

U

Ulyssa
Meaning: Walker
Origin: Greek

V

Vakila
Meaning: Truth
Origin: Arabic

Vale
Meaning: Lives in the valley
Origin: Latin

Valentina
Meaning: Strong and healthy
Origin: Latin

Valeria
Meaning: Strength
Origin: Latin

Valiqa
Meaning: Trustworthy
Origin: Arabic

Vanesia
Meaning: Butterfly
Origin: Greek

Vanya
Meaning: God Is Gracious
Origin: Slavic

Veda
Meaning: Knowledge or wisdom
Origin: Sanskrit

Velda
Meaning: Power, ruler
Origin: American

Velinda
Meaning: Beautiful
Origin: Italian

Verona
Meaning: Truth
Origin: Italian

Viera
Meaning: Truth
Origin: Latin

Violet
Meaning: Purple
Origin: Latin

Violette
Meaning: Purple
Origin: French

Viorica
Meaning: Bluebell
Origin: Romanian

Virginia
Meaning: Maiden
Origin: Latin

Viveka
Meaning: Wisdom
Origin: Indian

Vivian
Meaning: Lively
Origin: Latin

Vivianna
Meaning: Lively
Origin: Latin

Vivienne
Meaning: Lively
Origin: French

Vonda
Meaning: A wanderer
Origin: English

Vonnie
Meaning: Womanly, brave
Origin: Latin

W

Wanda
Meaning: Wanderer
Origin: German

Wanetta
Meaning: Pale-skinned
Origin: English

Wynonna
Meaning: First born daughter
Origin: Native American

X

Xandra
Meaning: Defender of the people
Origin: Greek

Xanthe
Meaning: Golden
Origin: Greek

Xanthia
Meaning: Yellow
Origin: Greek

Xarika
Meaning: Life blessing, princess
Origin: Arabic

Xavia
Meaning: Bright or splendid
Origin: Arabic

Xaviera
Meaning: Bright, splendid
Origin: Arabic

Xeanee
Meaning: The one that cannot be broken
Origin: Arabic

Xene
Meaning: Welcoming
Origin: Greek

Xenia
Meaning: Hospitable, welcoming
Origin: Greek

Xia
Meaning: Glow of the sunrise
Origin: Chinese

Ximena
Meaning: One who hears
Origin: Spanish

Xin
Meaning: Beautiful
Origin: Chinese

Xiomara
Meaning: Famous in battle
Origin: Spanish

Xochitl
Meaning: Flower
Origin: Aztec

Xoey
Meaning: Life
Origin: Greek

Y

Yadra
Meaning: Mother
Origin: Spanish

Yaima
Meaning: Water conduit
Origin: Argentine

Yakeera
Meaning: Beloved, precious
Origin: Hebrew

Yalissa
Meaning: A beautiful flower
Origin: Hebrew

Yalonda
Meaning: Violet flower
Origin: Spanish

Yana
Meaning: God is gracious
Origin: Hebrew

Yanika
Meaning: God is gracious
Origin: Hebrew

Yasmina
Meaning: A beautiful flower that shines
Origin: Arabic

Yasmine
Meaning: Flower
Origin: Arabic

Ye
Meaning: Light
Origin: Chinese

Yona
Meaning: Dove
Origin: Hebrew

Yonah
Meaning: Dove
Origin: Unknown

Yonita
Meaning: Dove
Origin: Hebrew

Yvonne
Meaning: Yew tree
Origin: French

Z

Zadie
Meaning: Prosperous, fortunate
Origin: Arabic

Zahara
Meaning: To shine, flower
Origin: Hebrew

Zandra
Meaning: Defender of mankind
Origin: Spanish

Zandria
Meaning: Ray of light
Origin: Greek

Zanetta
Meaning: God's gift
Origin: Spanish

Zara
Meaning: Radiance
Origin: Unknown

Zaria
Meaning: Derived from Sarah meaning princess
Origin: Hebrew

Zeena
Meaning: Beautiful
Origin: African

Zelda
Meaning: Strong woman
Origin: German

Zemira
Meaning: Song
Origin: Hebrew

Zemirah
Meaning: Joyous melody
Origin: Hebrew

Zemora
Meaning: Praised
Origin: Hebrew

Zena
Meaning: Belonging to Zeus
Origin: Greek

Zeva
Meaning: Wolf
Origin: Hebrew

Zira

Meaning: Messenger
Origin: Hebrew

Ziya

Meaning: Splendor, glow
Origin: Arabic

Zulema

Meaning: Peace
Origin: Hebrew

CLASSIC

"A good name will shine forever."

Girl ♀

A

Andy
Meaning: Manly
Origin: Greek

Ashley
Meaning: The Greek Goddess of wild animals
Origin: Greek

B

Becca
Meaning: To tie or bind
Origin: Hebrew

Beverley
Meaning: Woman from the beaver meadow
Origin: Old English

Bianca
Meaning: White
Origin: Italian

C

Catherine
Meaning: Pure
Origin: Greek

Cecil
Meaning: Blind
Origin: Latin

Charlotte
Meaning: Free
Origin: French

Charmaine
Meaning: Freeman, strong
Origin: English

Chantel
Meaning: Singer, to sing
Origin: African

Courtney
Meaning: From the court
Origin: English

D

Diana
Meaning: Divine
Origin: Greek

Diane
Meaning: Divine
Origin: Latin

Dionne
Meaning: Divine
Origin: Greek

G

Gemma
Meaning: Precious stone
Origin: Italian

Georgina
Meaning: Farmer
Origin: Greek

Geraldine
Meaning: Spear ruler
Origin: German

J

Jackie
Meaning: Likely derived from the name John meaning God is gracious
Origin: Hebrew

Jacqueline
Meaning: Supplanter
Origin: French

Jessica
Meaning: God beholds
Origin: Hebrew

Joe
Meaning: God will give
Origin: Hebrew

K

Karen
Meaning: Pure
Origin: Unknown

Katherine
Meaning: Pure
Origin: Greek

Keisha
Meaning: Her life, woman
Origin: American

L

Lianne/Leanne
Meaning: Grace
Origin: English

M

Marie
Meaning: Star of the sea
Origin: Latin

Mercy
Meaning: Merciful
Origin: English

N

Nadine
Meaning: Hope
Origin: French

Natalie
Meaning: Birthday of the Lord, Christmas Day
Origin: French/Latin

Natasha
Meaning: Born on Christmas day
Origin: Russian

Nicole
Meaning: Victory of people
Origin: Greek

O

Olivia
Meaning: Olive tree
Origin: Latin

P

Pearl
Meaning: Pearl
Origin: Unknown

Prudence
Meaning: Caution
Origin: Unknown

R

Rachel
Meaning: Ewe
Origin: Hebrew

Rebecca
Meaning: To bind
Origin: Hebrew

Rochelle
Meaning: Little Rock, rest
Origin: German

Rosemary
Meaning: Dew of the sea
Origin: Latin

Ryan
Meaning: Little king
Origin: Irish

S

Sharlene
Meaning: Free man or free woman
Origin: German

Shireen
Meaning: Sweet
Origin: Persian

Shirley
Meaning: Bright meadow
Origin: English

T

Tanya

Meaning: Fairy queen
Origin: Slavic

V

Vanessa

Meaning: Butterfly
Origin: Greek

Victoria

Meaning: Victory
Origin: Latin

RELIGIOUS

"Babies are a bit of stardust blown from the hands of God."

Girl ♀

A

Aaliyah
Meaning: Exalted
Origin: Arabic

Abelia
Meaning: Sigh, breath, vapour
Origin: Hebrew

Abigail
Meaning: Cause of joy
Origin: Hebrew

Abrianna
Meaning: Mother of many nations
Origin: Hebrew

Abrihet
Meaning: She shines
Origin: Hebrew

Adah
Meaning: Adornment
Origin: Hebrew

Adalia
Meaning: God is my refuge
Origin: Hebrew

Ahanti
Meaning: Eternal
Origin: Hindi

Aisha
Meaning: Alive and well
Origin: Arabic

Aliyah
Meaning: Exalted
Origin: Arabic

Amaris
Meaning: Promised by God
Origin: Hebrew

Anaya
Meaning: God has answered
Origin: Hebrew

Angel
Meaning: Messenger
Origin: Greek

Angela
Meaning: Heavenly messenger
Origin: Greek

Angelina
Meaning: Messenger
Origin: Italian

Angelique
Meaning: Messenger
Origin: French

Aniyah
Meaning: God favors
Origin: Hebrew

Arianna
Meaning: Most holy
Origin: Latin

Arie
Meaning: Lion of God
Origin: Hebrew

Arielle
Meaning: Lion of God
Origin: Hebrew

Azrael
Meaning: Helped by God
Origin: Hebrew

B

Belicia
Meaning: God is my oath
Origin: Spanish

Benecia
Meaning: Blessed one
Origin: Spanish

Brielle
Meaning: God is my strength
Origin: French

C

Camilla
Meaning: Religious helper
Origin: French

Camille
Meaning: Religious helper
Origin: french

Carmel
Meaning: Garden of God
Origin: Hebrew

Carmen
Meaning: Spanish form of Carmel meaning “garden of God”
Origin: Hebrew

Celeste
Meaning: Heavenly
Origin: Latin

Charisse
Meaning: Grace
Origin: French

Chinara
Meaning: May God receive
Origin: Nigerian

Chinue
Meaning: God's blessing
Origin: African–Nigeria

Christina
Meaning: Follower of Christ
Origin: Hebrew

Christine
Meaning: Follower of Christ
Origin: Hebrew

Chrystyna
Meaning: Follower of Christ
Origin: Greek

Cyrille
Meaning: Lord
Origin: Unknown

D

Damilola
Meaning: God has given me wealth
Origin: African

Dana
Meaning: God is my judge
Origin: Hebrew

Daniella
Meaning: God is my judge
Origin: Hebrew

Danita
Meaning: God will judge
Origin: Hebrew

Dashawna
Meaning: God is gracious
Origin: African American

Deon
Meaning: God
Origin: Greek

Domini
Meaning: Lord
Origin: Latin

Dominica
Meaning: Belonging to the Lord
Origin: Latin

Dominique
Meaning: Of the Lord
Origin: Latin

E

Eiliyah

Meaning: Beautiful one to grow in peace and love with God
Origin: Arabic

Eleasha

Meaning: God is salvation
Origin: Hebrew

Eliana

Meaning: God has answered
Origin: Hebrew

Elianna

Meaning: My God has answered
Origin: Hebrew

Elisha

Meaning: God is my salvation
Origin: Hebrew

Elissia

Meaning: God is my salvation
Origin: Hebrew

Elizabeth

Meaning: God is my oath
Origin: Hebrew

Ellone

Meaning: God loves me
Origin: African

Elly

Meaning: God is my light
Origin: Hebrew

Elsie

Meaning: My God is an oath
Origin: Hebrew

Elyse

Meaning: God's promise
Origin: Latin

Emna

Meaning: Believing
Origin: Arabic

Ezri

Meaning: My help
Origin: Hebrew

F

Faith
Meaning: Complete trust, devotion
Origin: English

G

Gabrielle
Meaning: God is my strength
Origin: Hebrew

Gayle
Meaning: Father's joy
Origin: Hebrew

Genesis
Meaning: The beginning
Origin: Greek

Gloria
Meaning: Glory
Origin: Latin

Glory
Meaning: Glory to God
Origin: English

Grace
Meaning: Charm, goodness, generosity
Origin: Latin

H

Hania
Meaning: Happy
Origin: Arabic

Haniel
Meaning: God's grace
Origin: Hebrew

Haskell
Meaning: God's helmet
Origin: Norse

I

Inaya
Meaning: God Answered
Origin: Hebrew

Isabella
Meaning: Devoted to God
Origin: Italian

Isobel
Meaning: God is oath
Origin: Hebrew

Ivria
Meaning: A Hebrew woman, from the land of Abraham
Origin: Hebrew

J

Jackie
Meaning: Likely derived from the name John meaning God is gracious
Origin: Hebrew

Jacquetta
Meaning: Supplanter
Origin: Hebrew/French

Jada
Meaning: The knowing one, wise
Origin: Hebrew

Jaden
Meaning: God has heard
Origin: Hebrew

Jana
Meaning: God is gracious
Origin: Hebrew

Janus
Meaning: Gateway
Origin: Latin

Jariah
Meaning: Tributary Lord
Origin: Hebrew

Jazz
Meaning: Derived from Jasmine meaning gift from God
Origin: Persian

Jesse
Meaning: The Lord exists
Origin: Hebrew

Jessica
Meaning: God beholds
Origin: Hebrew

Joelle
Meaning: Jehovah is God
Origin: Hebrew

Jojo
Meaning: God raises
Origin: Hebrew

Jordan
Meaning: Flowing down
Origin: Hebrew

Jordyn
Meaning: To flow down
Origin: Hebrew

K

Kalisa
Meaning: One who has given herself to God
Origin: American

Keshon
Meaning: God is merciful
Origin: English

Keziah
Meaning: Cassia tree
Origin: Hebrew

Kian
Meaning: God is Gracious
Origin: Irish

Kyra
Meaning: Lord
Origin: Greek

Kyrina
Meaning: Lord
Origin: Greek

L

Lasean
Meaning: God is gracious
Origin: American

Lashawna
Meaning: God's grace
Origin: American

Lashonda
Meaning: God is gracious
Origin: American

M

Machele
Meaning: Resembles God
Origin: Hebrew

Madihah
Meaning: Praiseworthy
Origin: Arabic

Makanaka
Meaning: God is good
Origin: African–Zimbabwe

Makayla
Meaning: Who is like God?
Origin: Hebrew

Mande
Meaning: God is within us
Origin: Hebrew

Mawusi
Meaning: In the hands of God
Origin: African–Ghana

Mekelle
Meaning: Who is like God?
Origin: African American

Michelle
Meaning: Who is like God?
Origin: French

Mikaili
Meaning: Who is like God?
Origin: African

Misha
Meaning: Who resembles God?
Origin: Hebrew

Mishon/Michonne
Meaning: A kind gift from the God
Origin: Hebrew

N

Nakimera
Meaning: Gift from God
Origin: African–Uganda

Natalie
Meaning: Birthday of the Lord / Christmas Day
Origin: French/Latin

Natasha
Meaning: Born on Christmas day
Origin: Russian

Nichelle
Meaning: Like God
Origin: Hebrew

Nkechi
Meaning: Gift of God
Origin: African

Noel
Meaning: Born on Christmas
Origin: French

Nokutenda
Meaning: By faith
Origin: African–Zimbabwe

Nuru
Meaning: Filled with light
Origin: African–Swahili

O

Onyeka
Meaning: God is the greatest
Origin: African–Nigeria

Ora
Meaning: Prayer
Origin: Latin

P

Pascal
Meaning: Easter
Origin: Latin/French

Paula
Meaning: Small, humble
Origin: Latin

Psalm
Meaning: Song
Origin: Greek

R

Ramla
Meaning: Prophetess
Origin: African–Swahili

Ranielle
Meaning: God is my judge
Origin: American/African

Rashawn
Meaning: God is gracious
Origin: Hebrew

Rashona
Meaning: God's favorite
Origin: American

Ruth

Meaning: Compassionate friend
Origin: Hebrew

S

Saint

Meaning: Holy person
Origin: American

Seanna

Meaning: God is gracious
Origin: Irish

Selasi

Meaning: God hears me
Origin: African

Shakeina

Meaning: God's presence
Origin: Hebrew

Shamica/Shamika

Meaning: Majestic
Origin: American

Shana

Meaning: God is gracious
Origin: Hebrew

Shauna/Shawna

Meaning: God is gracious
Origin: Irish

Shona

Meaning: God is gracious
Origin: Hebrew

Shonda

Meaning: God is gracious
Origin: American

Shontaya

Meaning: God is gracious
Origin: American

Simone

Meaning: God has heard
Origin: Hebrew

T

Teana

Meaning: Follower of Christ
Origin: English

Tendai

Meaning: Be thankful to God
Origin: African

Tiana
Meaning: Follower of Christ
Origin: English

Trinity
Meaning: Pertaining To The Holy Trinity of the Father, the Son, and the Holy Spirit
Origin: English

Tyann
Meaning: Follower of Christ
Origin: Latin

U

Ulyaa
Meaning: High, eminent
Origin: Arabic

Urice
Meaning: Light
Origin: Hebrew

X

Xami
Meaning: Praised
Origin: Hebrew

Y

Yanika
Meaning: God is gracious
Origin: Hebrew

Yosephina
Meaning: Derived from Joseph meaning God will multiply
Origin: Hebrew

Z

Zantina
Meaning: Little saint
Origin: Brazilian

BOYS' NAMES A-Z BY CATEGORY

POSITIVE MEANING

"Happiness is a mood. Positivity is a mindset."

Boy ♂

A

Ace
Meaning: Unity
Origin: Latin

Adeagbo
Meaning: Crown of the family
Origin: Nigerian

Adebisi
Meaning: The king or the crown
Origin: Unknown

Adewole
Meaning: The king
Origin: African

Adlan
Meaning: Fair, just
Origin: Arabic

Adunbi
Meaning: Pleasant
Origin: Nigerian

Aeneas
Meaning: Praised, praiseworthy
Origin: Latin

Ahanu
Meaning: He laughs
Origin: Native American

Ajani
Meaning: He fights for what he wants
Origin: Africa (Nigeria)

Akintunde
Meaning: The brave one
Origin: Nigerian

Akio
Meaning: Bright, luminous
Origin: Japanese

Akira
Meaning: Bright, intelligent, clear
Origin: Japanese

Akoni
Meaning: Too great to estimate
Origin: Hawaiian

Alan
Meaning: Handsome
Origin: Celtic

Allen
Meaning: Noble
Origin: Celtic

Amar

Meaning: Long life, immortal
Origin: Arabic

Ameer

Meaning: Prince, chief
Origin: Arabic

Amin

Meaning: Honest, faithful, trustworthy
Origin: Arabic

Amiri

Meaning: Prince
Origin: Arabic

Anthone

Meaning: Highly praised, priceless one
Origin: Latin

Anthony

Meaning: Worthy of praise
Origin: Latin

Antoine

Meaning: Derived from Anton meaning priceless
Origin: Latin

Antonio

Meaning: Worthy of praise
Origin: Latin

Antonne

Meaning: Priceless
Origin: Latin

Aron

Meaning: Moutain of strength
Origin: Greek

Arsenio

Meaning: Strong, virile
Origin: Greek

Askia

Meaning: The joy of greatness
Origin: African

Asma

Meaning: High status
Origin: Arabic

Austin

Meaning: Great
Origin: Unknown

B

Bali

Meaning: Strength
Origin: Indonesia

Barack

Meaning: Blessing
Origin: African

Baron
Meaning: Noble person
Origin: English

Bayo
Meaning: Joy
Origin: African

Beau
Meaning: Beautiful
Origin: French

Bernard
Meaning: Brave as a bear
Origin: Germanic

Bobby/Bobbie
Meaning: Famous, bright
Origin: German

Brendon
Meaning: Prince
Origin: Irish

C

Cairo
Meaning: Victorious
Origin: Arabic

Calix
Meaning: Handsome
Origin: Greek

Cara
Meaning: Beloved
Origin: Italian

Carim
Meaning: Generous
Origin: Arabic

Cavin
Meaning: Beautiful at birth
Origin: German

Cedric
Meaning: Chief
Origin: English

Chance
Meaning: Fortune
Origin: English

Chuma
Meaning: Wealthy
Origin: Egyptian

Clarence
Meaning: Bright, shining
Origin: Latin

Clement
Meaning: Gentle
Origin: English

Coman
Meaning: Noble
Origin: Arabic

D

Daevin
Meaning: Brilliant
Origin: Jamaican

Daevon
Meaning: Derived from Davon meaning beloved
Origin: Hebrew

Dakari
Meaning: Happiness, joy
Origin: African

Dandrae
Meaning: Strong, brave, courageous
Origin: Greek

Dandras
Meaning: Strong, brave, courageous
Origin: Greek

Danso
Meaning: One who can be trusted
Origin: African

Dante
Meaning: Lasting
Origin: Italian

Daran
Meaning: Great
Origin: Gaelic

Darik
Meaning: Ruler of the land
Origin: Old English

Dario
Meaning: Kingly
Origin: Italian

Darion
Meaning: Gift
Origin: Greek

Darius
Meaning: Upholder of the good
Origin: Persian

Darren
Meaning: Great
Origin: Irish

Dayo
Meaning: Happiness has come
Origin: African

Delroy
Meaning: The king
Origin: French

Demas
Meaning: Popular
Origin: Biblical

Denali
Meaning: Great one
Origin: Native American

Duke
Meaning: Leader
Origin: Latin

Duro
Meaning: Tough
Origin: Latin

E

Earl
Meaning: Noble man, warrior
Origin: English

Edmund
Meaning: Riches, wealthy protector
Origin: English

Edward
Meaning: Wealth, prosperous
Origin: Old English

Ekon
Meaning: Strong
Origin: African

Eldrick
Meaning: Sage ruler
Origin: Greek

Eli
Meaning: High, elevated
Origin: Hebrew

Elroy
Meaning: The king
Origin: French

Emerson
Meaning: Brave, powerful
Origin: British

Emile
Meaning: To excel
Origin: French

Eniola
Meaning: Wealthy person
Origin: African

Ephraim
Meaning: Very fruitful
Origin: Hebrew

Ernard
Meaning: Brave as a bear
Origin: German

Ezana
Meaning: Loving leader
Origin: African

Eze
Meaning: King
Origin: African

F

Fardeen
Meaning: One who has triple strength
Origin: Arabic

Farouk
Meaning: The one who knows right from wrong
Origin: Arabic

Fela
Meaning: Lucky
Origin: Latin

Felix
Meaning: Lucky
Origin: Latin

Frederick
Meaning: Peaceful ruler
Origin: German

Fritz
Meaning: Peaceful ruler
Origin: German

G

Gamba
Meaning: Warrior
Origin: African

Garon
Meaning: Guardian
Origin: French

Gene
Meaning: Born lucky
Origin: Greek

Ghalen
Meaning: Calm
Origin: Greek

Gonza
Meaning: Love
Origin: African

Grady
Meaning: Noble
Origin: Gaelic

Gyasi
Meaning: Wonderful
Origin: Egyptian

H

Habib
Meaning: Loved one
Origin: Arabic

Hakeem
Meaning: Wise
Origin: Arabic

Hasani
Meaning: Handsome
Origin: African

I

Ifeanyichukwu
Meaning: Nothing is impossible with God
Origin: African

Illario
Meaning: Cheerful, happy
Origin: Italian

Ilori
Meaning: Special treasure
Origin: African

Isaac
Meaning: He will laugh
Origin: Hebrew

Iyaaz
Meaning: Generous, bountiful
Origin: Arabic

J

Jahi
Meaning: Dignified
Origin: Swahili

Jai
Meaning: Champion
Origin: Sanskrit

Jarius
Meaning: To stand out and shine
Origin: Greek

Jayden
Meaning: Thankful
Origin: Unknown

Jaydene
Meaning: Thankful
Origin: Unknown

Jazz
Meaning: Derived from Jasmine meaning gift from God
Origin: Persian

Jenae
Meaning: God has answered
Origin: Unknown

Jibril/Jubril
Meaning: Angel
Origin: Arabic

Jimar
Meaning: Handsome
Origin: Arabic

Julius
Meaning: Youthful
Origin: Latin

Justin
Meaning: Fair, righteous
Origin: Latin

Justus
Meaning: Upright, just
Origin: Latin

K

Kalei
Meaning: The beloved
Origin: Hawaiian

Kalen
Meaning: Strong leader
Origin: Gaelic

Kamaal
Meaning: Perfection
Origin: Arabic

Kamari
Meaning: Great joy
Origin: American

Karim
Meaning: Generous
Origin: Arabic

Katlego
Meaning: Success
Origin: African

Kato
Meaning: All-knowing
Origin: Latin

Katungi
Meaning: Rich
Origin: African

Kay
Meaning: Pure
Origin: Unknown

Kayleb
Meaning: Faithful
Origin: Hebrew

Kayode
Meaning: He who brings joy
Origin: African

Kekoa
Meaning: Brave one
Origin: Hawaiian

Kendi
Meaning: The loved one
Origin: African

Kenji
Meaning: Intelligent, strong
Origin: Japanese

Kevin
Meaning: Handsome
Origin: Irish

Khalan
Meaning: A strong warrior
Origin: Arabic

Khari
Meaning: Kingly
Origin: Swahili

Kimani
Meaning: Adventurer
Origin: African

Kimoni
Meaning: A great man
Origin: African

Kinta
Meaning: Laughter
Origin: Aboriginal

Kioko
Meaning: Born with happiness
Origin: Japanese

Kirabo
Meaning: Gift from God
Origin: African

Kisembo
Meaning: Gift
Origin: African

Kota
Meaning: Happiness
Origin: Japanese

L

Lado
Meaning: Great or famous ruler
Origin: Georgian

Lakista
Meaning: One who is bold
Origin: American

Lareina
Meaning: The queen
Origin: Spanish

Latif
Meaning: Gentle, kind
Origin: Arabic

Lerato
Meaning: Song of my soul, to adore a person
Origin: African

Lolonyo
Meaning: Love is beautiful
Origin: African

Luca
Meaning: Light
Origin: Latin

Lucas
Meaning: Giver of light
Origin: Latin

Lucius
Meaning: Light
Origin: Latin

Lux
Meaning: Light
Origin: Latin

M

Maanan
Meaning: Very generous, bountiful
Origin: Arabic

Mabili
Meaning: The inspired one
Origin: African

Mack
Meaning: Greatest
Origin: Latin

Magezi
Meaning: Wise
Origin: African

Magic
Meaning: Full of wonder
Origin: American

Maia
Meaning: Great
Origin: Latin

Major
Meaning: Superior
Origin: Latin

Makami
Meaning: Beauty
Origin: Japanese

Makula
Meaning: Handsome
Origin: Sanskrit

Malawa
Meaning: Flourishing
Origin: African

Malik
Meaning: King
Origin: Arabic

Mandla
Meaning: Strength
Origin: African

Mansa
Meaning: Conqueror, king, king of kings
Origin: African

Marcel
Meaning: Young warrior
Origin: French

Mareke
Meaning: Beloved
Origin: Hebrew

Mariatu
Meaning: Pure
Origin: African

Marquis
Meaning: Nobleman
Origin: French

Masopha
Meaning: Chieftain, leader of the tribe
Origin: African–Basotho

Mfumu
Meaning: Leader, hero
Origin: African–Bakongo of Zaire

Mhina
Meaning: Delightful
Origin: African–Bakongo of Zaire

Milo
Meaning: Merciful
Origin: British

Mosego
Meaning: Blessings
Origin: African -Tswana

Moseph
Meaning: Blessed
Origin: African–Abua of Nigeria

Mugisa
Meaning: Blessing
Origin: African–Rutooro

Mukisa
Meaning: Good fortune or luck
Origin: African–Uganda

Mwai
Meaning: Success
Origin: African

Mwamba
Meaning: Strong, powerful
Origin: African

N

Neil
Meaning: Victory, champion
Origin: Irish

Nelson
Meaning: Champion
Origin: Gaelic

Neo/Neyo
Meaning: Gift
Origin: African Origin/American

Niall
Meaning: Champion
Origin: Irish

Nickoy
Meaning: Gifted child
Origin: Jamaican

Nile/Nyle
Meaning: Champion
Origin: Gaelic

Nirvan
Meaning: Bliss
Origin: Unknown

Nkosi
Meaning: King, ruler
Origin: African–Zulu

Nolan
Meaning: Noble, champion
Origin: Irish

Ntsako
Meaning: Joy, happiness
Origin: African–Tsonga of Central Africa

Nyack
Meaning: Won't Give Up
Origin: African

Nyall
Meaning: Champion
Origin: Unknown

O

Oba
Meaning: King
Origin: African–Nigeria

Obataiye
Meaning: King of the world
Origin: African–Nigeria

Ochieng
Meaning: Born when the sun shines
Origin: African

Odai
Meaning: Possibly derived from Uday meaning rise, ascend, to appear
Origin: Sanskrit

Ojore
Meaning: Warrior
Origin: African

Ola
Meaning: Wealth
Origin: African–Nigerian

Olatunde
Meaning: Wealth
Origin: African–Nigerian

Olaudah
Meaning: Vicissitude, fortune
Origin: African

Omari
Meaning: Flourishing
Origin: Arabic

Omorede
Meaning: A royal prince
Origin: African

Orlando
Meaning: Famous throughout the land
Origin: Unknown

Otis
Meaning: Rich, wealth, prosperous
Origin: English

Meaning: Wealth
Origin: German

P

Patrick
Meaning: Noble man
Origin: English

Phomello
Meaning: Succeed
Origin: African - South Africa

Prince
Meaning: Leader, first
Origin: Latin

Pruitt
Meaning: Brave little one
Origin: French

Q

Qabir
Meaning: Very good
Origin: Arabic

Qani
Meaning: Satisfied, content
Origin: Arabic

Qasit
Meaning: Just, fair
Origin: Arabic

Quinlan
Meaning: Very strong
Origin: Irish

R

Raanan
Meaning: Fresh, green, flourishing
Origin: Hebrew

Reagan
Meaning: Little king
Origin: Irish

Reese
Meaning: Enthusiastic
Origin: Welsh

Reilly
Meaning: Courageous
Origin: Irish

Rex
Meaning: King
Origin: Latin

Reymundo/ Reimundo
Meaning: Guards wisely
Origin: French

Rohan
Meaning: Ascending
Origin: Sanskrit

Ronald
Meaning: Ruler's counselor
Origin: Unknown

Royal
Meaning: The King
Origin: English

Rufaro
Meaning: Happiness
Origin: Africa-Zimbabwe

Runako
Meaning: Handsome
Origin: Africa-Zimbabwe

Russom
Meaning: One who is a leader
Origin: Swahili

Ryker
Meaning: Rich
Origin: German

S

Sage
Meaning: Wise
Origin: Old French

Sanyu
Meaning: Happiness
Origin: African

Saphir
Meaning: Sapphire, gem
Origin: Biblical

Sebahive
Meaning: Bearer of good fortune
Origin: African

Sebastian
Meaning: Venerable
Origin: Greek

Sekani
Meaning: Joy
Origin: African

Sekayi
Meaning: Laughter
Origin: African

Sekou
Meaning: Wise
Origin: African

Selam
Meaning: Peace
Origin: African

Sentwali
Meaning: Courageous
Origin: African

Shai
Meaning: Gift
Origin: Hebrew

Shakir
Meaning: Thankful
Origin: Unknown

Shan
Meaning: Wise
Origin: Indian

Shandon
Meaning: Wise
Origin: Gaelic

Shaquille
Meaning: Handsome
Origin: Arabic

Shay
Meaning: Admirable
Origin: Gaelic

Shingai
Meaning: Courageous
Origin: African

Shobi
Meaning: Glorious
Origin: Hebrew

Sihle
Meaning: Beautiful feeling
Origin: African

Sijuwade
Meaning: A man who is destined for greatness
Origin: African

Sipho
Meaning: Gift
Origin: African

Skylar
Meaning: Scholar
Origin: Dutch

Sterling
Meaning: Little star
Origin: English

Sudi
Meaning: Luck
Origin: African

Suhuba
Meaning: Friend
Origin: African

Sultan
Meaning: King
Origin: Arabic

T

Tadiwa
Meaning: We have been favored
Origin: African

Takeo
Meaning: Strong as bamboo
Origin: Japanese

Takudzwa
Meaning: We have been honored
Origin: African

Tapiwa
Meaning: Gift
Origin: African

Tariro
Meaning: Hope
Origin: African

Tashinga
Meaning: Perseverance
Origin: African

Tata
Meaning: Cheerful
Origin: Unknown

Taurean
Meaning: Strong
Origin: Latin

Tavon
Meaning: Nature
Origin: Scottish

Tene
Meaning: One who is much loved
Origin: African

Teneil
Meaning: Champion
Origin: American

Terrence
Meaning: Smooth
Origin: Latin

Terris
Meaning: Gracious
Origin: Latin

Terry
Meaning: Powerful
Origin: German

Teshi
Meaning: Cheerful
Origin: African

Tevin
Meaning: Beautiful at birth
Origin: American

Thabiti
Meaning: A genuine man
Origin: African

Thane
Meaning: Clan Chieftain
Origin: Scottish

Themba
Meaning: Trust
Origin: African

Tiwa
Meaning: One who owns the crown
Origin: African

Tlholo
Meaning: Victory
Origin: African

Tomi
Meaning: Rich
Origin: Japanese

Tony/Toni
Meaning: Worthy of praise
Origin: Latin

Tory
Meaning: Victory
Origin: English

Trayvon
Meaning: Brave one
Origin: American

Tsebo
Meaning: Knowledge
Origin: African

Tshepo
Meaning: Hope
Origin: African

Tumaini
Meaning: Hope
Origin: African

Tupac
Meaning: Royal
Origin: American

Tyrese
Meaning: Smooth
Origin: Latin

Tyrique
Meaning: Saver of the people
Origin: Unknown

Tyrus
Meaning: Strength
Origin: American

U

Umran
Meaning: Prosperity
Origin: Arabic

Unika
Meaning: Shine
Origin: African

Usain
Meaning: Likely derived from Husain meaning beautiful
Origin: Arabic

Uzo
Meaning: The Road is good
Origin: African

V

Vakar
Meaning: Respect, dignity
Origin: Arabic

Valerian
Meaning: Strong
Origin: Latin

Victor
Meaning: Winner, conqueror
Origin: Latin

Vinn
Meaning: Conqueror
Origin: English

Viyan
Meaning: Special knowledge
Origin: Indian

W

William
Meaning: Determined, resolute protector
Origin: English

Wylie
Meaning: Clever, crafty
Origin: Old English

X

Xaden
Meaning: Cleansing beam of Light
Origin: American

Xavion
Meaning: A fighter
Origin: African

Xerxes
Meaning: Ruler over heroes
Origin: Greek

Xho
Meaning: Leader
Origin: African

Y

Yafeu
Meaning: Bold
Origin: African–Fente

Yasir
Meaning: Rich
Origin: Arabic

Yerodin
Meaning: Studious
Origin: African–Congo

Z

Zahar/Zahir
Meaning: Shine, sparkle, bloom, flourishing
Origin: Arabic

Zahur
Meaning: Eminent
Origin: Arabic

Zaid

Meaning: Abundance, increase
Origin: Arabic

Zain

Meaning: Grace, beauty
Origin: Arabic

Zana

Meaning: Wise
Origin: Kurdish

Zebedee

Meaning: Abundant
Origin: Biblical

Zeeshan

Meaning: Magnificent
Origin: Arabic

Zen

Meaning: Meditation
Origin: Japanese

Zene

Meaning: Beautiful
Origin: African–Nigeria

Ziza

Meaning: Splendor, abundance
Origin: Biblical/Hebrew

Zohar

Meaning: Brilliance
Origin: Hebrew

Zyan

Meaning: Little king
Origin: English

SPACE & NATURE

"Shoot for the moon. Even if you miss, you'll land in the stars."

Boy ♂

A

Adan
Meaning: Earth or fire
Origin: Hebrew

Afi
Meaning: Fire
Origin: Polynesian

Alpine
Meaning: Fair
Origin: Latin

Apollo
Meaning: Destroyer
Origin: Greek

Archer
Meaning: Bowman. Also refers to the Sagittarius constellation
Origin: English

Arden
Meaning: Great forest
Origin: Latin

Arlo
Meaning: Fortified hill
Origin: English

Arun
Meaning: Dawn
Origin: Indian

Asahi
Meaning: Sunlight
Origin: Japanese

Ash
Meaning: Ash tree
Origin: British

Ashton
Meaning: Ash tree places
Origin: English

Aston
Meaning: From the East town
Origin: English

Astro
Meaning: One of the stars
Origin: Greek

Atlas
Meaning: Enduring
Origin: Greek

Azibo
Meaning: Earth
Origin: African

B

Blair
Meaning: Field, plain
Origin: Scottish

Blaze
Meaning: Flame
Origin: Latin

Bradley
Meaning: Broad meadow
Origin: English

Brook
Meaning: Water, stream
Origin: English

Brooklyn
Meaning: Beautiful brook
Origin: Unknown

Burleigh
Meaning: Meadow with knotty-trunk trees
Origin: Old English

C

Callum
Meaning: Dove
Origin: Scottish

Canyon
Meaning: Footpath
Origin: Spanish

Cedar
Meaning: Cedar tree
Origin: American

Chane
Meaning: Oak-hearted
Origin: French

Citana
Meaning: Star in the sky
Origin: Native American

Clayton
Meaning: Town built on clay
Origin: English

Cleavant
Meaning: From the cliff
Origin: Greek

Cleveland
Meaning: From the cliff
Origin: English

Clevon
Meaning: From the cliff
Origin: English

Clifton
Meaning: Town by the cliff
Origin: English

Clinton
Meaning: From the town on a hill
Origin: English

Conan
Meaning: Little wolf
Origin: Celtic

Cornel
Meaning: A tree
Origin: Latin

Cyrus
Meaning: Sun
Origin: Unknown

D

Dalton
Meaning: From the valley town
Origin: Old English

Damani
Meaning: Tomorrow
Origin: American

Deimos
Meaning: One of the moons of Mars
Origin: Greek

Deiondre
Meaning: Valley
Origin: American

Delmar
Meaning: Of the sea
Origin: Spanish

Derry
Meaning: Oak grove
Origin: Irish

Diron
Meaning: Bird
Origin: American

Douglas
Meaning: Dark stream
Origin: Scottish

Dylan
Meaning: Son of the sea
Origin: Welsh

E

Eilon
Meaning: Oak tree
Origin: Hebrew

Elan
Meaning: Tree
Origin: Hebrew

Elio
Meaning: Derived from Helios meaning sun
Origin: Spanish

Elon
Meaning: Oak tree
Origin: Hebrew

Ennis
Meaning: Island
Origin: Irish

Everest
Meaning: Dweller from the Eure river. Also, the tallest mountain in the world.
Origin: English

F

Florin
Meaning: Flower
Origin: Latin

Ford
Meaning: River crossing
Origin: British

Forest
Meaning: Woodsman, woods
Origin: French

G

Galaxy
Meaning: Large system of stars
Origin: American

Gelso
Meaning: Mulberry tree
Origin: Italian

Geo
Meaning: Earth
Origin: Greek

George
Meaning: Farmer
Origin: Greek

H

Hamza
Meaning: Lion
Origin: Arabic

Hawke
Meaning: Hawk
Origin: English

Hayden
Meaning: Hay valley
Origin: English

Heath
Meaning: Heathland dweller
Origin: English

Heathcliff
Meaning: Cliff near a heath
Origin: British

Helal
Meaning: First moon
Origin: Arabic

I

Idra
Meaning: Fig tree
Origin: Hebrew

Ilan
Meaning: Tree
Origin: Hebrew

Ilani
Meaning: My tree
Origin: Hebrew

Ishaan
Meaning: The Sun
Origin: Indian

Ixia
Meaning: South African flower
Origin: African

J

Jacy
Meaning: The Moon
Origin: Native American

Jericho
Meaning: City of moons
Origin: Arabic

Juno
Meaning: Youth. Also, a NASA space probe orbiting Jupiter
Origin: Latin

Jupiter
Meaning: Supreme God. Also the largest planet in our solar system
Origin: Latin

K

Kai
Meaning: Sea
Origin: Hawaiian

Kaia
Meaning: The sea
Origin: Hawaiian

Kaito
Meaning: Ocean
Origin: Unknown

Kamar
Meaning: Moon
Origin: Arabic

Kauri
Meaning: Tree
Origin: Maori

Knox
Meaning: Round-top hill
Origin: British

L

Laikin
Meaning: Body of water
Origin: English

Lake
Meaning: Body of water
Origin: British

Laken
Meaning: From the lake
Origin: English

Lamar
Meaning: Of the sea
Origin: German

Lincoln
Meaning: From the lake settlement
Origin: English

Linden
Meaning: Made from Linwood, lime tree
Origin: English

Lovell
Meaning: Wolf
Origin: French

M

Madzimoyo
Meaning: Water of life
Origin: African

Marlon
Meaning: Little hawk
Origin: French

Marlow
Meaning: Driftwood
Origin: British

Maxwell
Meaning: Great stream
Origin: Scottish

Meadow
Meaning: Field of grass
Origin: American

Moana
Meaning: Ocean, sea
Origin: Hawaiian

Molapo
Meaning: River, stream
Origin: African–Basotho

Murphy
Meaning: Sea warrior
Origin: Irish

Musoke
Meaning: Rainbow
Origin: African

N

Nahele
Meaning: Forest
Origin: Native American

Nash
Meaning: Dweller by the ash tree
Origin: English

Nevis
Meaning: Snow
Origin: Spanish

Nile
Meaning: Champion. Also the longest river in Africa.
Origin: Irish

Nimbus
Meaning: Resembling a rain cloud
Origin: Latin

Nodin
Meaning: Wind
Origin: Native American

North
Meaning: North
Origin: British

O

Oakley
Meaning: Meadow of oak trees
Origin: English

Ocean
Meaning: Sea
Origin: Greek

Ohio
Meaning: Great river
Origin: Native American

Oliver
Meaning: Olive tree
Origin: French

Orion
Meaning: Rising in the sky
Origin: Greek

Orson
Meaning: Bear cub
Origin: Latin

P

Pacific
Meaning: Tranquil
Origin: Portuguese

Parker
Meaning: Keeper of the park
Origin: English

Pelabo
Meaning: Lightning
Origin: Arabic

Phoenix
Meaning: Dark red
Origin: Greek

Piers
Meaning: Rock
Origin: Unknown

Q

Qamar
Meaning: Moon
Origin: Arabic

Quesnel
Meaning: From the little oak tree
Origin: French

R

Ranger
Meaning: Guardian of the forest
Origin: French

Ray
Meaning: Beam of light
Origin: British

Reid
Meaning: Red
Origin: Scottish

Ren
Meaning: Lotus
Origin: Japanese

Rhodes
Meaning: Where roses grow
Origin: German

Rhys
Meaning: Fire
Origin: Welsh

Rio
Meaning: River
Origin: Spanish

River
Meaning: Stream of water that flows to the sea
Origin: English

Rocket
Meaning: A jet propelled tube
Origin: English

Rowan
Meaning: Rowan tree
Origin: English

Ruby
Meaning: A deep red precious stone
Origin: Latin

S

Safari
Meaning: Journey
Origin: African

Sango
Meaning: Coral
Origin: Japanese

Satima
Meaning: Young bull
Origin: African

Sidney
Meaning: Wide meadow
Origin: English

Silas
Meaning: Forest
Origin: Latin

Soleil
Meaning: Sun
Origin: French

Star
Meaning: Luminous astronomical object
Origin: Greek

Sterling
Meaning: Little Star
Origin: English

Stormy
Meaning: Impetuous nature
Origin: American

Sunni
Meaning: Sunshine
Origin: English

Suriya
Meaning: Sun
Origin: Unknown

Sydel/Sidell
Meaning: From the wide valley
Origin: English

T

Tamal
Meaning: A tree with a very dark bark
Origin: Indian

Tamar
Meaning: Date
Origin: Hebrew

Theros
Meaning: Summer
Origin: Greek

Timber
Meaning: Wood
Origin: English

Trent
Meaning: Gushing waters
Origin: Latin

U

Udayna
Meaning: Rising sun
Origin: Sanskrit

Udgama
Meaning: Rising star
Origin: Sanskrit

Umakanta
Meaning: Moonlight
Origin: Sanskrit

V

Vance
Meaning: Marshland
Origin: English

W

Wainani
Meaning: Beautiful water
Origin: Hawaiian

Walden
Meaning: Wooded valley
Origin: English

Winter
Meaning: Cold season
Origin: American

Woody
Meaning: From the lane in the wood
Origin: American

X

Xylo
Meaning: Wood, forest
Origin: Greek

Y

Yardley
Meaning: Enclosed meadow
Origin: English

Z

Zait
Meaning: Olive
Origin: Hebrew

Zenith
Meaning: Highest point
Origin: English

Zephyr
Meaning: West wind
Origin: Greek

Zeren
Meaning: Golden
Origin: Arabic

Zoran
Meaning: Derived from Zora meaning Dawn
Origin: Arabic

AFRICAN ORIGIN

"If we stand tall, it's because we stand on the shoulders of our ancestors." -African Proverb

Boy ♂

A

Abayomi
Meaning: My enemies tried to mock me but God didn't allow them
Origin: African–Nigerian

Abeeku
Meaning: Born on Wednesday
Origin: African–Ghana

Abejide
Meaning: Born during winter
Origin: African–Nigeria

Abiade
Meaning: Born of royal parents
Origin: African–Nigeria

Abibola
Meaning: Born wealthy
Origin: African

Abidemi
Meaning: Child born during father absence
Origin: African

Abu
Meaning: Nobility, popularity
Origin: African

Achan
Meaning: Trouble maker
Origin: African–Ugandan

Achebe
Meaning: One that is protected by God
Origin: African–Nigeria

Addae
Meaning: Morning sun
Origin: African–Ghana

Addo
Meaning: King of the path
Origin: African

Ade
Meaning: Crown, royal
Origin: African

Adeagbo
Meaning: Crown of the family
Origin: African–Nigeria

Adeben
Meaning: Twelfth born
Origin: African

Adebisi
Meaning: The king or the crown
Origin: African

Adejola
Meaning: The crown needs honor
Origin: African

Adewole
Meaning: The king
Origin: African

Adio
Meaning: He is righteous
Origin: African

Adisa
Meaning: One who is clear
Origin: African

Adjatay
Meaning: Prince
Origin: African–Cameroon

Adjo
Meaning: Righteous
Origin: African -Nigeria

Adofo
Meaning: The warrior
Origin: African–Ghana

Adunbi
Meaning: Pleasant
Origin: Nigerian

Adwin
Meaning: An artist, creative person
Origin: African–Ghana

Afolabi
Meaning: Born in wealth and high status
Origin: African–Nigeria

Afram
Meaning: A river in Ghana
Origin: African

Africa
Meaning: From Africa
Origin: African

Agu
Meaning: Having the agility and strength of a leopard
Origin: African–Nigeria

Agyei
Meaning: Messenger from God
Origin: African–Ghana

Agyeman
Meaning: Fourteenth born
Origin: African–Ghana

Ajani
Meaning: He fights for what he wants
Origin: African

Ajayi
Meaning: Born face down
Origin: African

Akande
Meaning: First born
Origin: African–Nigeria

Akanni
Meaning: To bring wealth, possession, profits
Origin: African

Akia
Meaning: First born
Origin: African–Uganda

Akiiki
Meaning: A good friend
Origin: African–Uganda

Akintunde
Meaning: The brave one
Origin: African

Akono
Meaning: It is my turn
Origin: African

Akuchi
Meaning: Wealth from God
Origin: African

Akwasi
Meaning: Born on Sunday
Origin: African

Alake
Meaning: One to be honored
Origin: African

Amadi
Meaning: Rejoicing
Origin: African

Amare
Meaning: Handsome
Origin: African–Ethopia

Amari
Meaning: Strength
Origin: African

Amazu
Meaning: No one knows everything
Origin: African

Ambakisye
Meaning: God has been merciful
Origin: African

Ametefe
Meaning: Born after father's death
Origin: African

Ampah
Meaning: Trust
Origin: African–Ghana

Amri
Meaning: Power
Origin: African

Andwele
Meaning: God brings me
Origin: African–Tanzania

Anesu
Meaning: God is with us
Origin: African–Zimbabwe

Asante
Meaning: Thank you
Origin: African

Ashaki
Meaning: Beautiful
Origin: African

Askia
Meaning: The joy of greatness
Origin: African

Ayinde
Meaning: We gave praises and he came
Origin: African

Ayo
Meaning: Happiness, joy
Origin: African

Ayubu
Meaning: Whoever perseveres
Origin: African

Azibo
Meaning: Earth
Origin: African

Azikiwe
Meaning: Full of vigor
Origin: African

B

Babafemi
Meaning: My father loves me
Origin: African

Badru
Meaning: Born at full moon
Origin: African–Swahili

Bahari
Meaning: Sea man
Origin: African

Bahati
Meaning: Luck
Origin: Swahili

Bakari
Meaning: Promising
Origin: African

Bako
Meaning: Guest
Origin: African

Banga
Meaning: Sword
Origin: African

Banji
Meaning: Second born twin
Origin: African

Barack
Meaning: Blessing
Origin: African

Baruti
Meaning: Teacher
Origin: African

Bayo
Meaning: Joy
Origin: African

Belay
Meaning: Superior
Origin: African

Bem
Meaning: Peace
Origin: African

Biton
Meaning: Born after a long wait
Origin: African

Bomani
Meaning: Warrior
Origin: African

C

Camara
Meaning: Teacher
Origin: African

Chabwera
Meaning: Finally arrived
Origin: African

Changa
Meaning: Strong as iron
Origin: African

Chata
Meaning: Ending
Origin: African

Chenzira
Meaning: Born while traveling
Origin: African

Chetachi
Meaning: Remember God
Origin: African

Chiamaka
Meaning: God is beautiful
Origin: African

Chiazam
Meaning: Answer from God
Origin: African

Chibale
Meaning: Kinsman
Origin: African–Egypt

Chicha
Meaning: Beloved
Origin: African–Swahili

Chidubem
Meaning: Guided by God
Origin: African

Chiemeka
Meaning: God has performed great deeds
Origin: African

Chijioke
Meaning: Divinity gives talent
Origin: African

Chika
Meaning: Divinity is the greatest
Origin: African

Chike
Meaning: Power of God
Origin: African

Chikelu
Meaning: Created by God
Origin: African

Chikere
Meaning: Created by God
Origin: African

Chikezie
Meaning: Well made by God
Origin: African

Chikwendu
Meaning: May God give you life
Origin: African

Chima
Meaning: God knows
Origin: African

Chimelu
Meaning: Made of God
Origin: African

Chinelo
Meaning: Thoughts of God
Origin: African

Chinyelu
Meaning: God gave
Origin: African–Nigeria

Chioke
Meaning: Gift of God
Origin: African–Nigeria

Chioma
Meaning: God is good, great
Origin: African

Chiumbo
Meaning: A small creation
Origin: African

Congo
Meaning: A country in Africa–The Democratic Republic of Congo
Origin: African

D

Dakarai
Meaning: Rejoice
Origin: African

Dakari
Meaning: Happiness, joy
Origin: African

Danjuma
Meaning: Born on Friday
Origin: African

Danladi
Meaning: Born on Sunday
Origin: African

Danso
Meaning: One who can be trusted
Origin: African

Daren
Meaning: Born at night
Origin: African

Daudi
Meaning: Beloved one
Origin: African

Dayo
Meaning: Happiness has come
Origin: African

Deka
Meaning: Pleasing
Origin: African

Dele
Meaning: Come home
Origin: African

Dembe
Meaning: Peace
Origin: African

Diara
Meaning: Gift
Origin: African

Dingiswayo
Meaning: One in distress. Also a great Zulu chief.
Origin: African

Djimon
Meaning: Powerful blood
Origin: African

Dumi
Meaning: The inspirer
Origin: African

E

Ebere
Meaning: One who shows mercy
Origin: African

Ehioze
Meaning: Stands above envy
Origin: African

Eintou
Meaning: Pearls of wisdom
Origin: African

Ekene
Meaning: Praise
Origin: African

Ekon
Meaning: Strong
Origin: African

Eniola
Meaning: Wealthy person
Origin: African

Ermias
Meaning: God will uplift
Origin: African

Essien
Meaning: 6th born
Origin: African

Ezana
Meaning: Loving leader
Origin: African

Eze
Meaning: King
Origin: African

Ezeamaka
Meaning: One who is splendid as a king
Origin: African

Ezenachi
Meaning: The king rules
Origin: African

Ezeoha
Meaning: A people's king
Origin: African

Ezinwene
Meaning: Good brothers/ good sisters
Origin: African

F

Fabunni
Meaning: God has given me this
Origin: African

Farai
Meaning: Rejoice, be happy
Origin: African

Femi
Meaning: Love me
Origin: African

Feneku
Meaning: Born past term
Origin: African

Fenyang
Meaning: Victor, conqueror
Origin: African

Fisseha
Meaning: Happiness, joy
Origin: African

Foluke
Meaning: Under God's protection
Origin: African

G

Gamba
Meaning: Warrior
Origin: African

Garai
Meaning: To be settled
Origin: African

Godana
Meaning: Male child
Origin: African

Gonza
Meaning: Love
Origin: African

Gwinyai
Meaning: To have strength
Origin: African

Gyasi
Meaning: Wonderful
Origin: African–Egypt

H

Habimana
Meaning: God exists
Origin: African

Hamisi
Meaning: Born on Thursday
Origin: African

Hasani
Meaning: Handsome
Origin: African

I

Idowu
Meaning: Born after twins
Origin: African

Ifeancho
Meaning: The desired child
Origin: African

Ifeanyichukwu
Meaning: Nothing is impossible with God
Origin: African

Ifoma
Meaning: A good thing, beautiful
Origin: African

Iggi
Meaning: Only son
Origin: African

Ikechukwu
Meaning: The strength of God
Origin: African

Ikenna
Meaning: Father's power
Origin: African

Ilo
Meaning: Sunshine
Origin: African

Ilori
Meaning: Special treasure
Origin: African

Imarogbe
Meaning: Born to a good family
Origin: African

J

Ja
Meaning: Magnetic
Origin: African

Jabilo
Meaning: Medicine man
Origin: African

Jabulani
Meaning: He who rejoices
Origin: African

Jafaru
Meaning: Brook, creek
Origin: African

Jahi
Meaning: Dignified
Origin: African-Swahili

Jaja
Meaning: Gift of God
Origin: African

Jawara
Meaning: Lover of peace
Origin: African

Jayvyn
Meaning: Light spirit
Origin: African

Jenue
Meaning: From Jenue in Nigeria
Origin: African

Jibade
Meaning: Related to royalty
Origin: African

Jibri
Meaning: Angel of Allah
Origin: African

Jimiyu
Meaning: Born during summer
Origin: African

Jirani
Meaning: Neighbor
Origin: African-Swahili

Jomo
Meaning: Flaming Spear
Origin: African-Swahili

Juma
Meaning: Born on Friday
Origin: African

Jumaane
Meaning: Born on Tuesday
Origin: African

Jumoke
Meaning: Everyone loves the child
Origin: African

K

Kabelo
Meaning: To share
Origin: African

Kabili
Meaning: Brave
Origin: African

Kabonero
Meaning: A sign or symbol
Origin: African

Kabonesa
Meaning: Difficult birth
Origin: African

Kafele
Meaning: Worth giving one's life for
Origin: African

Kagiso
Meaning: Peace
Origin: African

Kairu
Meaning: Black one
Origin: African

Kamau
Meaning: Quiet warrior
Origin: African

Kame
Meaning: Desolate, arid
Origin: African

Kanelo
Meaning: Enough
Origin: African

Kanoro
Meaning: Sword sharpener
Origin: African

Kapeni
Meaning: Knife
Origin: African

Karume
Meaning: Master
Origin: African–Swahili

Kaseko
Meaning: Mock, ridicule
Origin: African

Kashka
Meaning: A friendly man
Origin: African

Kassa
Meaning: Reparation, compensation
Origin: African

Katlego
Meaning: Success
Origin: African

Katungi
Meaning: Rich
Origin: African

Kayode
Meaning: He who brings joy
Origin: African

Kayonga
Meaning: Ash
Origin: African

Kazi
Meaning: Work
Origin: African

Keb
Meaning: Earth
Origin: African

Kehinde
Meaning: Secondborn of twins
Origin: African

Keita
Meaning: Blessing
Origin: African

Kendi
Meaning: The loved one
Origin: African

Kenyatta
Meaning: Musician
Origin: African

Kenyi
Meaning: Boy born after 3 or more girls
Origin: African

Khamisi
Meaning: Born on Thursday
Origin: African

Khari
Meaning: Kingly
Origin: Swahili

Kiano
Meaning: The wizard tools
Origin: African

Kifimbo
Meaning: Very thin child
Origin: African

Kijana
Meaning: Youth
Origin: African

Kimani
Meaning: Adventurer
Origin: African

Kimoni
Meaning: A great man
Origin: African

Kimotho
Meaning: Left-handed
Origin: African

Kione
Meaning: Someone who comes from nowhere
Origin: African

Kirabo
Meaning: Gift from God
Origin: African

Kisembo
Meaning: Gift
Origin: African

Kitoko
Meaning: Beautiful
Origin: African

Kitwana
Meaning: Pledge to live
Origin: African–Swahili

Kofi
Meaning: Born on a Friday
Origin: African

Kojo
Meaning: Born on a Monday
Origin: African

Kontar
Meaning: Only child
Origin: African

Kwabena
Meaning: Born on Tuesday
Origin: African

Kwada
Meaning: Night has fallen
Origin: African

Kwame
Meaning: Born on a Saturday
Origin: African

Kwanza
Meaning: Beginning, birth. An annual holiday celebrated by Black people
Origin: African–Swahili

Kwasi
Meaning: Born on Sunday
Origin: African

Kwayera
Meaning: Dawn
Origin: African

L

Lebron
Meaning: King
Origin: African

Lehana
Meaning: One who refuses
Origin: African

Lerato
Meaning: Song of my soul, to adore a person
Origin: African

Lereko
Meaning: Abundance, merciful
Origin: African

Lolonyo
Meaning: Love is beautiful
Origin: African

M

Mabili
Meaning: The inspired one
Origin: African

Mablevi
Meaning: Do not deceive
Origin: African

Madzimoyo
Meaning: Water of life
Origin: African

Magezi
Meaning: Wise
Origin: African

Magomu
Meaning: Younger of twins
Origin: African

Maitho
Meaning: The eyes that give you sight
Origin: African

Makalani
Meaning: Clerk
Origin: African

Makalo
Meaning: Wonder, surprise
Origin: African

Makondo
Meaning: War
Origin: African

Malawa
Meaning: Flourishing
Origin: African

Mandla
Meaning: Strength
Origin: African

Mansa
Meaning: Conqueror, king, king of kings
Origin: African

Mariatu
Meaning: Pure
Origin: African

Masamba
Meaning: Leaves
Origin: African

Masego
Meaning: Blessings
Origin: African

Mashaka
Meaning: Trouble
Origin: African

Mashama
Meaning: You are surprised
Origin: African

Masiko
Meaning: Hope
Origin: African

Masimba
Meaning: Power
Origin: African–Zimbabwe

Masopha
Meaning: Chieftain, leader of the tribe
Origin: African–Basotho

Mawuli
Meaning: There is a God
Origin: African–Ghana

Mbiya
Meaning: Money, wealth
Origin: African

Mbizi
Meaning: Water
Origin: African–Egypt

Mensah
Meaning: Born third
Origin: African

Mfumu
Meaning: Leader, hero
Origin: African

Mhina
Meaning: Delightful
Origin: African

Mikaili
Meaning: Who is like God?
Origin: African

Minana
Meaning: Miracle
Origin: African–Bantu of Zimbabwe

Minkah
Meaning: Justice
Origin: African

Molapo
Meaning: River, stream
Origin: African–Basotho

Mongo
Meaning: Famous
Origin: African–Nigerian

Morathi
Meaning: Wise man
Origin: African–Kikuyu of Kenya

Moreri
Meaning: Preacher
Origin: African

Morocco
Meaning: A country in Africa
Origin: African

Mosego

Meaning: Blessings
Origin: African–Tswana

Moseph

Meaning: Blessed
Origin: African–Abua of Nigeria

Mosi

Meaning: The first born
Origin: African

Moyo

Meaning: Heart
Origin: African–Zimbabwe

Mufaro

Meaning: Happiness
Origin: African–Zimbabwe

Mugisa

Meaning: Blessing
Origin: African

Mukisa

Meaning: Good fortune or luck
Origin: African

Mukundi

Meaning: Victor
Origin: African–Bantu of Zimbabwe

Munashe

Meaning: With God
Origin: African–Zimbabwe

Musoke

Meaning: Rainbow
Origin: African

Mwai

Meaning: Success
Origin: African

Mwaka

Meaning: Born at the beginning of the year
Origin: African

Mwamba

Meaning: Strong, powerful
Origin: African

Mwinyi

Meaning: King
Origin: African–Swahili

N

Najja
Meaning: Born after
Origin: African

Nalo
Meaning: Loveable
Origin: African

Namib
Meaning: Vast place
Origin: African

Nangwaya
Meaning: One who will not be trifled with
Origin: African

Naserian
Meaning: The lucky one
Origin: African

Nathi
Meaning: God is with us
Origin: African–Zulu

Natine
Meaning: Of the Natine tribe
Origin: African

Ndale
Meaning: Cheat, a trick
Origin: African

Ndidi
Meaning: Patience
Origin: African–Nigeria

Ndoki
Meaning: Sorcerer
Origin: African

Ndulu
Meaning: Dove
Origin: African–Nigeria

Ngoni
Meaning: Mercy
Origin: African–Zimbabwe

Nkosi
Meaning: King, ruler
Origin: African

Ntsako
Meaning: Joy, happiness
Origin: African

Nwa
Meaning: Son
Origin: African–Nigeria

Nyabera
Meaning: The good one
Origin: African–Luo of Kenya

Nyack
Meaning: Won't give up, tenacity
Origin: African

Nyamekye
Meaning: God's gift
Origin: African–Ghana

O

Oba

Meaning: King
Origin: African–Nigeria

Obadele

Meaning: The king arrives
Origin: African–Nigeria

Obafemi

Meaning: The king loves me
Origin: African–Nigeria

Obama

Meaning: Bending, leaning
Origin: African–Luo of Kenyan

Obataiye

Meaning: King of the world
Origin: African–Nigeria

Obiajulu

Meaning: My heart is at peace
Origin: African–Nigeria

Ochieng

Meaning: Born when the sun shines
Origin: African

Odion

Meaning: First of twins
Origin: African

Ogochukwu

Meaning: The favor of God
Origin: African–Nigeria

Ojore

Meaning: Warrior
Origin: African

Okal

Meaning: To cross
Origin: African

Okoth

Meaning: Born when it was raining
Origin: African

Ola

Meaning: Wealth
Origin: African–Nigeria

Oladele

Meaning: Honor, wealth has come home
Origin: African–Nigeria

Olafemi

Meaning: Honor favors me
Origin: African–Nigeria

Olajuwon

Meaning: Wealth and honor are God's gifts
Origin: African–Nigeria

Olaniyan

Meaning: Respected
Origin: African–Nigeria

Olatunde
Meaning: Wealth
Origin: African–Nigeria

Olaudah
Meaning: Vicissitude, fortune
Origin: African

Olu
Meaning: God
Origin: African

Olubayo
Meaning: Highest delight
Origin: African–Nigeria

Olushola
Meaning: God has blessed or honored me
Origin: African–Nigeria

Oluyemi
Meaning: God has given me satisfaction
Origin: African–Nigeria

Omorede
Meaning: A royal prince
Origin: African

Onaedo
Meaning: Gold
Origin: African–Nigeria

Oratilwe
Meaning: Loved one
Origin: African

Osahar
Meaning: God hears me
Origin: African

Osakwe
Meaning: The Lord agrees
Origin: African

Osayaba
Meaning: The Lord forgives
Origin: African

Osaze
Meaning: Loved by God
Origin: African–Nigeria

Osei
Meaning: Noble or honorable
Origin: African–Ghana

Oya
Meaning: Wind warrior Goddess
Origin: African

P

Paolosi
Meaning: Little one
Origin: African–Basotho

Paseka
Meaning: Easter, born on Easter
Origin: African–Sesotho

Pelumi

Meaning: God is with me
Origin: African–Nigeria

Penda

Meaning: Love
Origin: African–Swahili

Phomello

Meaning: Succeed
Origin: African–South Africa

Polo

Meaning: Alligator
Origin: African

Q

Quashie

Meaning: Born on Sunday
Origin: African

R

Rafiki

Meaning: Friend
Origin: African

Rashidi

Meaning: Thinker, counselor
Origin: African

Reon

Meaning: Descendant of the king
Origin: African–South Africa

Reth

Meaning: King
Origin: African

Roho

Meaning: Soul
Origin: African

Rudo

Meaning: Love
Origin: Africa–Zimbabwe

Rufaro

Meaning: Happiness
Origin: Africa–Zimbabwe

Runako

Meaning: Handsome
Origin: Africa–Zimbabwe

Russom

Meaning: One who is a leader
Origin: African–Swahili

Rutendo

Meaning: Faith
Origin: Africa–Zimbabwe

S

Sabiti
Meaning: Born on Sunday
Origin: African

Sabola
Meaning: Pepper
Origin: African–Egypt

Sadiki
Meaning: Faithful
Origin: African

Safari
Meaning: Journey
Origin: African

Saidi
Meaning: Helper
Origin: African

Salako
Meaning: Born covered in membrane
Origin: African

Sandile
Meaning: You have increased our family
Origin: African

Sanyu
Meaning: Happiness
Origin: African

Sarki
Meaning: Chief
Origin: African

Satima
Meaning: Young bull
Origin: African

Sebahive
Meaning: Bearer of good fortune
Origin: African

Sekani
Meaning: Joy
Origin: African

Sekayi
Meaning: Laughter
Origin: African

Sekou
Meaning: Wise
Origin: African

Selam
Meaning: Peace
Origin: African

Selasi
Meaning: God hears me
Origin: African

Sentwali
Meaning: Courageous
Origin: African

Shaka
Meaning: Name given to the Chief of the Zulu tribe
Origin: African

Shingai
Meaning: Courageous
Origin: African

Shomari
Meaning: Forceful
Origin: African

Shumba
Meaning: Lion
Origin: African

Sihle
Meaning: Beautiful feeling
Origin: African

Sijuwade
Meaning: A man who is destined for greatness
Origin: African

Simba
Meaning: Lion
Origin: African

Sipho
Meaning: Gift
Origin: African

Sisi
Meaning: Born on Sunday
Origin: African

Siyolo
Meaning: Joy of Earth
Origin: African

Sudi
Meaning: Luck
Origin: African

Suhuba
Meaning: Friend
Origin: African

T

Tabansi
Meaning: One who endures
Origin: African

Tadiwa
Meaning: We have been favored
Origin: African

Tadiwanashe
Meaning: We are loved by God
Origin: African

Tafara
Meaning: We are happy
Origin: African

Taiwo

Meaning: First twin to taste the world
Origin: African

Takudzwa

Meaning: We have been honored
Origin: African

Tamuka

Meaning: We have risen
Origin: African

Tapiwa

Meaning: Gift
Origin: African

Tariro

Meaning: Hope
Origin: African

Tashinga

Meaning: Perseverance
Origin: African

Taye

Meaning: He has been seen
Origin: African

Temi (Temiloluwa)

Meaning: Mine
Origin: African

Tene

Meaning: One who is much loved
Origin: African

Teshi

Meaning: Cheerful
Origin: African

Thabiti

Meaning: A genuine man
Origin: African

Thando

Meaning: Love
Origin: African

Themba

Meaning: Trust
Origin: African

Thulani/Tulani

Meaning: Be quiet or be still
Origin: African

Tinashe

Meaning: God is with us
Origin: African

Tiwa

Meaning: One who owns the crown
Origin: African

Tiyamike

Meaning: We praise
Origin: African

Tlholo

Meaning: Victory
Origin: African

Toure
Meaning: Belonging to the Soussou or Maninka
Origin: African

Tsebo
Meaning: Knowledge
Origin: African

Tshepo
Meaning: Hope
Origin: African

Tumaini
Meaning: Hope
Origin: African

Tumo
Meaning: Fame
Origin: African

Twia
Meaning: Born after twins
Origin: African

Tyehimba
Meaning: We stand as a nation
Origin: African

U

Uba
Meaning: Lord
Origin: African

Uchenna
Meaning: God's thoughts
Origin: African

Unika
Meaning: Shine
Origin: African

Useni
Meaning: Testimony
Origin: African

Uzo
Meaning: The road is good
Origin: African

Uzoma
Meaning: Good way
Origin: African

W

Wafula
Meaning: Born during the rainy season
Origin: African–Kenya

Wakili
Meaning: Lawyer, representative
Origin: African

Wambua
Meaning: Born during the rainy season
Origin: African

Wasaki
Meaning: The enemy
Origin: African

X

Xavion
Meaning: A fighter
Origin: African

Xho
Meaning: Leader
Origin: African

Xola
Meaning: Stay in peace
Origin: African–Xhosa of South Africa

Y

Yafeu
Meaning: Bold
Origin: African–Fente

Yao
Meaning: Born on Thursday
Origin: African–Ghana

Yaro
Meaning: Son
Origin: African–Hausa of West Africa

Yawo
Meaning: Born on Thursday
Origin: African

Yenge
Meaning: Work
Origin: African–Mende of Sierra Leone

Yerodin
Meaning: Studious
Origin: African–Congo

Yohance

Meaning: God's gift
Origin: African–Hausa of West Africa

Z

Zaci

Meaning: God of fatherhood
Origin: African

Zaire

Meaning: The river that swallows other rivers
Origin: African

Zareb

Meaning: Guardian
Origin: African

Zawadi

Meaning: Gift
Origin: African–Swahili

Zene

Meaning: Beautiful
Origin: African–Nigeria

Zesiro

Meaning: First born of twins
Origin: African

Zo

Meaning: Spiritual leader
Origin: African

Zoan

Meaning: Departure
Origin: African

Zuberi

Meaning: Strong
Origin: African–Swahili

Zulu

Meaning: Heaven. The Zulu Kingdom was a powerful kingdom in Southern Africa in the 1800s. Today the Zulu people are the largest group in South Africa
Origin: African–South Africa

Zuva

Meaning: Day
Origin: African–Bantu of Zimbabwe

BIBLICAL

"A good name is more to be desired than great wealth."—*Proverbs 22:1*

Boy ♂

A

Aaron
Meaning: Exalted
Origin: Hebrew

Abda
Meaning: Servitude
Origin: Arabic

Abel
Meaning: Breath
Origin: Hebrew

Abiram
Meaning: My Father is exalted
Origin: Hebrew

Achaicus
Meaning: A native of Achaia
Origin: Greek

Adaiah
Meaning: Adornment of God
Origin: Hebrew

Adam
Meaning: Son of the red Earth
Origin: Hebrew

Adiel
Meaning: Ornament of God
Origin: Hebrew

Adio
Meaning: He is righteous
Origin: African

Adriel
Meaning: The flock of God
Origin: Hebrew

Aenon
Meaning: A fountain
Origin: Biblical

Ahaziah
Meaning: Vision of the Lord
Origin: Hebrew

Alijah
Meaning: The Lord is my God
Origin: Hebrew

Azariah
Meaning: Helped by God
Origin: Hebrew

B

Baal
Meaning: Lord
Origin: Hebrew

Ben
Meaning: Son of my right hand
Origin: Hebrew

Benjamin
Meaning: Son of my right hand
Origin: Hebrew

Benji
Meaning: Son of my right hand
Origin: Hebrew

C

Cain
Meaning: Spear
Origin: Hebrew

Cainan
Meaning: Possessor
Origin: Hebrew

Caiphas
Meaning: He that seeks with diligence
Origin: Biblical

Caleb
Meaning: Faithful
Origin: Hebrew

Calvary
Meaning: Skull
Origin: Biblical

Canaan
Meaning: Merchant, trader
Origin: Biblical

Carpus
Meaning: Fruit, fruitful
Origin: Biblical

Carshena
Meaning: A lamb
Origin: Biblical

Caspar
Meaning: Keeper of the treasure
Origin: Persian

Cephas
Meaning: A rock
Origin: Aramaic

Cesar
Meaning: Head of hair
Origin: Spanish

D

Dan
Meaning: God is my judge
Origin: Hebrew

Daniel
Meaning: God is my judge
Origin: Hebrew

David
Meaning: Beloved
Origin: Hebrew

Demas
Meaning: Popular
Origin: Biblical

Demetrius
Meaning: Earth
Origin: Greek

E

Eden
Meaning: Place of pleasure
Origin: Hebrew

Eli
Meaning: High, elevated
Origin: Hebrew

Elijah
Meaning: Yahweh is my God
Origin: Hebrew

Enoch
Meaning: Dedicated
Origin: Hebrew

Ephraim
Meaning: Very fruitful
Origin: Hebrew

Esaia
Meaning: God saves
Origin: Hebrew

Ethan
Meaning: Firm, strong
Origin: Hebrew

Ezekiel
Meaning: God will strengthen
Origin: Hebrew

Ezra
Meaning: Helper
Origin: Hebrew

F

Felix
Meaning: Lucky
Origin: Latin

G

Gabriel
Meaning: God is my strength
Origin: Hebrew

Galilee
Meaning: Wheel
Origin: Hebrew

H

Hananiah
Meaning: Grace
Origin: Hebrew

Hanniel
Meaning: Grace of God
Origin: Hebrew

Harran
Meaning: A singing
Origin: Hebrew

Henoch
Meaning: Dedicated
Origin: Hebrew

I

Immanuel
Meaning: God is with us
Origin: Hebrew

Iram
Meaning: Shining
Origin: Arabic

Isaac
Meaning: He will laugh
Origin: Hebrew

Iscah
Meaning: To behold
Origin: Hebrew

Israel
Meaning: May God prevail
Origin: Unknown

J

Jacob
Meaning: Supplanter
Origin: Hebrew

James
Meaning: Supplanter, replacer
Origin: Hebrew

Jared
Meaning: He descends
Origin: Hebrew

Javan
Meaning: Youth
Origin: Arabic

Jean-Jacques
Meaning: Equivalent to John James meaning God is gracious / supplanter
Origin: French

Jesse
Meaning: The Lord exists
Origin: Hebrew

Jevonte
Meaning: Son of Japheth
Origin: African American

Joel
Meaning: Jehovah is the Lord
Origin: Hebrew

John
Meaning: God is gracious
Origin: Hebrew

Jonah
Meaning: Dove
Origin: Unknown

Jonathan
Meaning: God's gift
Origin: Hebrew

Joseph
Meaning: God increases
Origin: Hebrew

Joshua
Meaning: The Lord is my salvation
Origin: Hebrew

Josiah
Meaning: God supports, heals
Origin: Hebrew

K

Kabzeel
Meaning: God gathers
Origin: Hebrew

Kadmiel
Meaning: Who stands before God
Origin: Hebrew

Kemuel
Meaning: Helper of God
Origin: Hebrew

Kenan
Meaning: Possession
Origin: Hebrew

L

Lazarus
Meaning: God has helped
Origin: Hebrew

Levi
Meaning: Joined
Origin: Hebrew

Lubin
Meaning: Heart of a man
Origin: Hebrew

Luke
Meaning: From Lucania
Origin: Greek

M

Mark
Meaning: Warlike, hammer, defender
Origin: Italian

Micah
Meaning: Who is like God?
Origin: Hebrew

Moses
Meaning: To draw out (of water)
Origin: Hebrew

N

Naaman
Meaning: Pleasant
Origin: Hebrew

Nehemiah
Meaning: God has comforted
Origin: Hebrew

Noah
Meaning: Rest, comfort
Origin: Hebrew

O

Obadiah
Meaning: Servant of God
Origin: Hebrew

Obed
Meaning: Servant of God
Origin: Hebrew

Ohad
Meaning: Loved one
Origin: Hebrew

P

Paul
Meaning: Small, humble
Origin: Latin

Peter
Meaning: Stone, rock
Origin: Greek

Philip
Meaning: Lover of horses
Origin: Greek

R

Raamah
Meaning: God's thunder
Origin: Hebrew

Rapha
Meaning: God who heals
Origin: Hebrew

Rephaiah
Meaning: Refreshment of the Lord
Origin: Hebrew

Reuben
Meaning: Behold a son
Origin: Hebrew

S

Salah
Meaning: Mission
Origin: Biblical

Samson
Meaning: Bright as the sun
Origin: Hebrew

Samuel
Meaning: God has heard
Origin: Hebrew

Saphir
Meaning: Sapphire, gem
Origin: Biblical

Sardis
Meaning: Prince of joy
Origin: Biblical

Shem
Meaning: Name
Origin: Hebrew

Shiloh
Meaning: Tranquil
Origin: Hebrew

Simeon
Meaning: God has heard
Origin: Hebrew

T

Taralah
Meaning: Strength
Origin: Biblical

Tarsus
Meaning: Winged, feathered
Origin: Biblical

Thaddeus
Meaning: Courageous heart
Origin: Aramaic

Thomas
Meaning: Twin
Origin: Aramaic

Timothy
Meaning: Honored by God
Origin: Greek

U

Uel
Meaning: Desiring God
Origin: Biblical

Uri
Meaning: My light
Origin: Hebrew

Urijah
Meaning: God is my light
Origin: Hebrew

Uzal
Meaning: Wandering
Origin: Biblical

V

Vaniah
Meaning: Nourishment
Origin: Biblical

Vophsi
Meaning: Fragrant
Origin: Hebrew

Z

Zaavan
Meaning: Trembling
Origin: Biblical

Zaccheus
Meaning: Pure, clean
Origin: Hebrew

Zachariah
Meaning: God remembers
Origin: Hebrew

Zacharias
Meaning: The Lord has remembered
Origin: Hebrew

Zebadiah
Meaning: Gift From God
Origin: Hebrew

Zebedee
Meaning: Abundant
Origin: Biblical

Zebediah
Meaning: Gift from God
Origin: Hebrew

Zechariah
Meaning: Memory of the Lord
Origin: Hebrew

Zedekiah
Meaning: The Lord is my justice
Origin: Hebrew

Zenas
Meaning: Hospitable
Origin: Greek

Zephaniah
Meaning: God has hidden
Origin: Hebrew

Zerahiah
Meaning: The Lord rising
Origin: Biblical

Ziba
Meaning: Army, strength
Origin: Biblical

Zion
Meaning: Highest place
Origin: Hebrew

Ziza
Meaning: Splendor, abundance
Origin: Hebrew

Zoar
Meaning: Little, small
Origin: Biblical

Zohar
Meaning: Brilliance
Origin: Hebrew

Zuriel
Meaning: Rock or strength of God
Origin: Hebrew

INFLUENTIAL PEOPLE

"I don't know who you will be but I know you will be my everything."

Boy ♂

A

Alexander

Meaning: Defender of men
Origin: Greek
Influential Person: Alexander Twilight – First African American to graduate from college.

Alton

Meaning: Old town
Origin: English
Influential Person: Alton Ellis – Jamaican singer and songwriter. Often labeled the Godfather of Rocksteady.

Amiri

Meaning: Prince
Origin: Arabic
Influential Person: Amiri Baraka – Award-winning writer of poetry, drama, fiction, and essays.

Arthur

Meaning: Bear
Origin: Celtic
Influential Person: Arthur Ashe – The only Black man to win Wimbledon (as of 2021) and the first Black tennis player to win 3 Grand Slam titles.

Ashanti

Meaning: The name of a tribe in Ghana
Origin: Greek
Influential Person: Ashanti Douglas – Award-winning singer, songwriter, and actress.

Askia

Meaning: The joy of greatness
Origin: African
Influential Person: Askia The Great – Great leader of the Songhai Empire in Western Africa.

Aubrey

Meaning: Ruler of The Elves, wise
Origin: French
Influential Person: Aubrey Graham aka Drake – Grammy award-winning rapper, actor, and entreprencur.

B

Barack

Meaning: Blessing
Origin: African
Influential Person: Barack Obama – 1st African American President of the USA.

Ben/Benjamin

Meaning: Son of my right hand
Origin: Hebrew
Influential Person: Benjamin O. Davis Jr – The first Black brigadier general in the US Air Force.

Bill

Meaning: Derived from William meaning resolute protector
Origin: English
Influential Person: Bill Russell – First Black coach in the NBA and the first to win an NBA Championship.

Bobby/Bobbie

Meaning: Famous, bright
Origin: German
Influential Person: Bobbie Brown – Grammy award-winning singer and rapper.

Bobby Marshall – First Black footballer in the NFL (along with Fritz Pollard)

Booker

Meaning: Maker of books
Origin: English
Influential Person: Booker T. Washington – America author, advisor to presidents, and civil rights activist.

Busta

Meaning: Dude
Origin: Jamaican
Influential Person: Busta Rhymes – Award-winning rapper.

C

Chance

Meaning: Fortune
Origin: English
Influential Person: Chance The Rapper (Chancelor Johnathan Bennett) – Grammy award-winning rapper.

Charlie

Meaning: Freeman
Origin: Old German
Influential Person: Bobby Marshall – First Black footballer in the NFL (along with Fritz Pollard).

Colin

Meaning: Young man
Origin: Gaelic
Influential Person: Colin Kaepernick - Influential civil rights activist and NFL quarterback.

Crispus

Meaning: Curly-haired
Origin: Latin
Influential Person: Crispus Attucks - Sailor, stevedore, and generally regarded as the first American killed in the American Revolution.

Curtis

Meaning: Courteous
Origin: English
Influential Person: Curtis Jackson aka 50 Cent - Rapper, entrepreneur, and TV producer.

D

Damon

Meaning: To tame
Origin: Greek
Influential Person: Damon Wayans - Stand-up comedian, writer, actor, and TV producer.

Daniel

Meaning: God is my judge
Origin: Hebrew
Influential Person: Daniel Hale Williams - General surgeon who performed the first successful heart surgery. Also, the founder of the first Black-owned hospital in the USA.

Daymond

Meaning: Bright
Origin: English
Influential Person: Daymond John - American businessman, investor, and TV personality.

Denzel

Meaning: From the high stronghold
Origin: English
Influential Person: Denzel Washington - Academy Award-winning actor, director, and producer.

Deontay

Meaning: Derived from Deon meaning belongs to God
Origin: Greek
Influential Person: Deontay Wilder – Former heavyweight boxing champion of the world.

Desmond

Meaning: Gracious defender
Origin: Irish
Influential Person: Desmond Tutu – South African activist, religious leader, and Nobel Prize winner.

Donell

Meaning: World ruler
Origin: Scottish
Influential Person: Donell Jones – American singer and songwriter.

Doris

Meaning: Gift
Origin: Greek
Influential Person: Doris Miller – The first Black American to be awarded the Navy Cross.

Drake

Meaning: Dragon
Origin: English
Influential Person: Drake – Canadian Grammy award-winning rapper, songwriter, and entrepreneur.

E

Eddie

Meaning: Wealthy guardian
Origin: English
Influential Person: Eddie Murphy – Award-winning actor, writer, producer, and considered one of the greatest stand-up comedians of all time.

Edward

Meaning: Wealth, prosperous
Origin: Old English
Influential Person: Edward Bouchet – The first Black person to receive a Ph.D. from any American university.

Emmett

Meaning: Universal
Origin: German
Influential Person: Emmett Till – A 14-year-old African American who was brutally murdered in Mississippi in 1955, after being accused of offending a white woman in a grocery store. Till posthumously became an icon of the civil rights movement.

Ermias

Meaning: God will rise/ God will uplift
Origin: African
Influential Person: Ermias Ashgedom aka Nipsey Hussle – American rapper & entrepreneur.

Ezana

Meaning: Loving leader
Origin: African
Influential Person: King Ezana of Aksum – Ruler of Askum (a region made up of modern-day Ethiopia and Eritrea). Aksum was the first Christian kingdom in Africa.

F

Fela

Meaning: Lucky
Origin: Latin
Influential Person: Fela Kuti – Multi-instrumentalist, composer, civil rights activist, and the pioneer of Afrobeats.

Forest

Meaning: Woodsman, woods
Origin: French
Influential Person: Forest Whitaker – Academy award-winning actor, director, and producer.

Frederick

Meaning: Peaceful ruler
Origin: German
Influential Person: Frederick Douglass – The leading campaigner against slavery in his time. He was a speaker, best-selling author and acted as an advisor to several presidents.

Fritz

Meaning: Peaceful ruler
Origin: German
Influential Person: Fritz Pollard – First Black Footballer in the NFL (along with Bobby Marshall).

G

Garrett

Meaning: Strong spear
Origin: Anglo-Saxon
Influential Person: Garrett Morgan – Inventor of the three-point traffic light system that we use today.

Garvey

Meaning: Rough peace
Origin: Gaelic
Influential Person: Marcus Garvey – Jamaican activist, entrepreneur, and orator for Black Nationalism and Pan-Africanism.

George

Meaning: Farmer
Origin: Greek
Influential Person: George Washington Carver – Born into slavery, he became a foremost botanist who advised world leaders on agriculture and nutrition.

George Foreman – Former boxing heavyweight champion of the world, successful businessman, and creator of the Foreman Grill.

J

Jack

Meaning: Likely derived from the name John meaning God is gracious
Origin: Hebrew
Influential Person: Jack Johnson – First Black boxing heavyweight champion of the world.

Jackie

Meaning: Likely derived from the name John meaning God is gracious
Origin: Hebrew
Influential Person: Jackie Robinson – First Black player in Major League Baseball, winner of the National League Most Valuable Player award, and civil rights activist.

Jaden

Meaning: God has heard
Origin: Hebrew
Influential Person: Jaden Smith – American rapper and actor. Son of Will Smith and Jada Pinkett-Smith.

James

Meaning: Supplanter, replacer
Origin: Hebrew
Influential Person: James Baldwin – Leader in the Civil Rights Movement.

Jason

Meaning: Healer
Origin: Greek
Influential Person: Jason Derulo – Award-winning singer, dancer, and songwriter.

Jean-Jacques

Meaning: Equivalent to John James meaning God is gracious / supplanter
Origin: French
Influential Person: Jean-Jacques Dessalines – In 1803, he defeated the last of Napoleon's forces and proclaimed independence for Haiti. Haiti was the first Black independent republic of which Dessalines was the first ruler.

Jean-Michel

Meaning: God is gracious
Origin: Hebrew
Influential Person: Jean-Michel Basquiat – American artist and the most financially successful African-American artist in history (at the time of writing).

Jermaine

Meaning: Brother
Origin: Latin
Influential Person: Jermaine Dupree – Award-winning record producer, rapper, and entrepreneur.

Jesse

Meaning: The Lord exists
Origin: Hebrew
Influential Person: Jesse Owens – 4 times Olympic gold medallist and the most successful athlete at the 1936 Berlin Olympics (held in Germany when under Hitler's rule).

Jimi

Meaning: Supplanter
Origin: Hebrew
Influential Person: Jimi Hendrix – Award-winning musician, singer, and songwriter. Hendrix is described by the Rock and Roll Hall of Fame as the "greatest instrumentalist in the history of rock music."

Joe

Meaning: God will give
Origin: Hebrew
Influential Person: Joe Louis – Professional boxer who is widely regarded as one of the best and most influential of all time.

John

Meaning: God is gracious
Origin: Hebrew
Influential Person: John Lewis – Leader in the Civil Rights Movement.

John Carlos – Famously displayed the Black Power salute at the 1968 Olympics when standing on the podium to accept the Bronze medal he had won for the 200m.

Jordan

Meaning: Flowing down
Origin: Hebrew
Influential Person: Jordan Peele – Actor, comedian, and filmmaker. He was the first Black director to win an Academy Award for Best Original Screenplay.

Jupiter

Meaning: Supreme God. Also the largest planet in our solar system
Origin: Latin
Influential Person: Jupiter Hammon – Born into slavery, Jupiter became a poet and the first Black American to have a poem published.

K

Keenan

Meaning: Ancient
Origin: Irish
Influential Person: Keenan Ivory Wayans – American actor, comedian, and filmmaker.

Kendrick

Meaning: Greatest champion/Bold ruler
Origin: Welsh
Influential Person: Kendrick Lamar – Grammy award-winning rapper, songwriter, and record producer.

Kevin

Meaning: Handsome
Origin: Irish
Influential Person: Kevin Hart – American comedian and actor; he is the highest-earning comedian of all time (as of 2021).

Kingsley

Meaning: From the King's meadow
Origin: English
Influential Person: Kingsley Junior Coman – French professional Footballer.

Kobe

Meaning: God will protect
Origin: Hebrew
Influential Person: Kobe Bryant – American basketballer and widely regarded as one of the greatest of all time.

Kwame

Meaning: Born on a Saturday
Origin: African
Influential Person: Kwame Nkrumah – First president of Ghana following its independence in 1960.

Kyrie

Meaning: Lord
Origin: Greek
Influential Person: Kyrie Irving – American basketballer.

L

Langston

Meaning: Tall man's town
Origin: English
Influential Person: Langston Hughes – American poet, novelist, and social activist.

Lebron

Meaning: King
Origin: African
Influential Person: Lebron James – Basketball player, widely considered one of the greatest of all time.

Lewis

Meaning: Famed warrior
Origin: English
Influential Person: Lewis Hamilton – British Formula 1 Driver and the first Black man to win an F1 championship.

Lewis Howard Latimer – Inventor, engineer, and writer; he invented the carbon filament which allowed a lightbulb to last longer.

Lionel

Meaning: Lion
Origin: Latin
Influential Person: Lionel Richie – Grammy award-winning singer, songwriter, and record producer.

M

Magic

Meaning: Full of wonder
Origin: American
Influential Person: Earvin "Magic" Johnson – American professional basketball player who is widely considered the best point guard of all time.

Malcolm

Meaning: Devotee of Saint Columba
Origin: Gaelic
Influential Person: Malcolm X – Civil rights activist and leader in the US Civil Rights Movement.

Mansa

Meaning: Conqueror, king, king of kings
Origin: African
Influential Person: Mansa Musa – One of the greatest African rulers of all time, Mansa Musa led the Mali Empire at the height of its power.

Marcus

Meaning: Follower of Mars (Roman God of war)
Origin: Latin
Influential Person: Marcus Garvey – Jamaican activist, entrepreneur, and orator for Black Nationalism and Pan-Africanism.

Martin

Meaning: Servant Of Mars (Roman God Of war)
Origin: Latin
Influential Person: Martin Luther King Jr. – Civil rights activist and the most prolific leader of the Civil Rights Movement in the USA.

Marvin

Meaning: Lives by the sea
Origin: Welsh
Influential Person: Marvin Gaye – Singer and songwriter who helped shape the sound of Motown in the 1960s.

Michael

Meaning: Who is like God?
Origin: Hebrew
Influential Person: Michael Jordan – Basketball player and businessman, widely considered the greatest basketball player of all time.

Michael Jackson – Award-winning artist, the King of Pop, and one of the best-selling artists of all time with more than 400m records sold worldwide.

Michael Omari aka Stomzy – One of the UK's most successful artists and the first Grime artist to have a #1 album in the UK.

Mongo

Meaning: Famous
Origin: African-Nigerian
Influential Person: Mongo Santamaria – Cuban percussionist and leading figure in the Pachanga and Boogaloo dance crazes of the 1960s.

Morgan

Meaning: Sea
Origin: Welsh
Influential Person: Morgan Freeman – Academy Award-winning actor.

Muhammad

Meaning: Praiseworthy
Origin: Arabic
Influential Person: Muhammad Ali – One of the greatest sportspeople of all time, he was boxing heavyweight champion of the world.

N

Neil

Meaning: Victory/Champion
Origin: Irish
Influential Person: Neil deGrasse Tyson – American astrophysicist, planetary scientist, and author.

Nelson

Meaning: Champion
Origin: Gaelic
Influential Person: Nelson Mandela – South African anti-apartheid revolutionary, political leader, and philanthropist who served as the first president of South Africa from 1994 to 1999.

Neo/Neyo

Meaning: Gift
Origin: African Origin/American
Influential Person: Ne-Yo (Shaffer Smith) – Grammy Award-winning singer and songwriter.

Nile/Nyle

Meaning: Champion
Origin: Gaelic
Influential Person: Nile Rogers – Grammy award-winning guitarist and songwriter. He has written, produced, and performed on albums that have sold more than 500m units worldwide.

O

Obama

Meaning: Bending, leaning
Origin: African–Luo of Kenyan
Influential Person: Barack Obama – 1st African American President of the USA.

Olaudah

Meaning: Vicissitude, fortune
Origin: African
Influential Person: Olaudah Equiano – Kidnapped and enslaved as a child from Benin (modern-day Nigeria), Olaudah dedicated his life to abolishing slavery and his autobiography had a powerful impact on public opinion around it.

Omari

Meaning: Flourishing
Origin: Arabic
Influential Person: Omari Hardwick – American actor.

Omarion

Meaning: Flourishing
Origin: Arabic
Influential Person: Omarion (Omari Grandberry) – An award-winning singer, songwriter, and lead singer of the band B2K.

Otis

Meaning: Rich, wealth, prosperous
Origin: English
Influential Person: Otis Redding – Grammy award-winning artist. Widely considered one of the greatest singers in American popular music history.

P

Percy

Meaning: One who pierces the valley
Origin: French
Influential Person: Percy Julian – Civil rights activist, chemist, and pioneer of synthesis of medicine from plants.

Q

Quincy

Meaning: Born fifth/fifth
Origin: French/Latin
Influential Person: Quincy Jones – Award-winning record producer, composer, and songwriter. He was the first African American to be musical director and conductor of the Academy Awards and he was the first African American to be nominated for an Academy Award for Best Original Song (along with Bob Russell).

R

Ralph

Meaning: Wolf counsel
Origin: English/German
Influential Person: Ralph Abernathy – Civil rights activist.

Ray

Meaning: Beam of light
Origin: British
Influential Person: Ray Charles – Grammy award-winning singer, songwriter, pianist, and pioneer of Soul music.

Romare

Meaning: Derived from Latin meaning a citizen of Rome
Origin: Latin
Influential Person: Romare Bearden – American artist, author, and songwriter.

Ruby

Meaning: A deep red precious stone
Origin: Latin
Influential Person: Ruby Bridges – The first Black student to attend the all-White William Frantz Elementary school at the height of desegregation.

S

Sean

Meaning: God is gracious
Origin: Irish
Influential Person: Sean Paul – Grammy award-winning Jamaican Dancehall artist.

Sean Combs – Grammy award-winning music producer, rapper, and businessman.

Shaka

Meaning: Name given to the Chief of the Zula tribe
Origin: African
Influential Person: Shaka Zulu – A strong and skilled chief of the Zulu empire.

Shaquille

Meaning: Handsome
Origin: Arabic
Influential Person: Shaquille O'Neal – American basketball player, regarded as one of the greatest of all time.

Shawn

Meaning: God is gracious
Origin: Irish
Influential Person: Shawn Carter (aka Jay Z) – American songwriter, rapper, and businessman. He has sold more than 125m records worldwide and was the first rapper to become a billionaire.

Sidney

Meaning: Wide meadow
Origin: English
Influential Person: Sidney Poitier – The first Black actor to win an Academy Award.

Spike

Meaning: A long heavy nail
Origin: English
Influential Person: Spike Lee – Award-winning film director.

Stephen

Meaning: Crown
Origin: Greek
Influential Person: Stephen Curry – American basketball player, regarded as one of the greatest point guards in history.

Sterling

Meaning: Little star
Origin: English
Influential Person: Raheem Sterling – English (Jamaican born) professional footballer.

Steve

Meaning: Crown
Origin: Greek
Influential Person: Steve Harvey – Presenter, actor, and best-selling author.

T

Ta-Nehisi

Meaning: Nubian
Origin: Egyptian
Influential Person:
Ta-Nehisi Coates – American author and journalist.

Terrence

Meaning: Smooth
Origin: Latin
Influential Person: Terrence Howard – Influential American Actor.

Thando

Meaning: Love
Origin: African
Influential Person: Thando Thabethe – South African actress and TV personality.

Tiger

Meaning: Powerful cat
Origin: American
Influential Person: Tiger Woods – American professional golfer and widely considered one of the greatest of all time.

Tommie

Meaning: Innocence
Origin: Hebrew
Influential Person: Tommie Smith – Famously displayed the Black Power salute at the 1968 Olympics when standing on the podium to accept the Gold medal he had won for the 200m.

Tory

Meaning: Victory
Origin: English
Influential Person: Tory Lanez (Daystar Peterson) – Award-winning Canadian rapper.

Toure

Meaning: Belonging to the Soussou or Maninka
Origin: African
Influential Person: Yaya Toure – Ivorian professional footballer.

Toussaint

Meaning: All saints
Origin: French
Influential Person: Toussaint L'Ouverture – Great military leader, he led a successful slave rebellion against colonial rule.

Trayvon

Meaning: Brave one
Origin: American
Influential Person: Trayvon Martin – An African American teenager who was shot dead whilst walking home. The term Black Lives Matter was first used in response to the acquittal of the man who shot him.

Trevor

Meaning: Big village
Origin: English
Influential Person: Trevor McDonald – Award-winning renowned British newsreader.

Trevor Noah – Emmy award-winning South African comedian, TV host, and political commentator.

Trey

Meaning: Three
Origin: English
Influential Person: Trey Songz (Tremaine Neverson) – American singer and songwriter.

Tupac

Meaning: Royal
Origin: American
Influential Person: Tupac Amaru Shakur – American rapper and widely considered one of the most influential of all time.

Tyehimba

Meaning: We stand as a nation
Origin: African
Influential Person: Tyehimba Jess – Pulitzer Prize for Poetry winner.

Tyler

Meaning: Maker of tiles
Origin: English
Influential Person: Tyler Perry – American Director, producer, and screenwriter and one of Time Magazine's Most Influential People (2020).

Tyrese

Meaning: Smooth
Origin: Latin
Influential Person: Tyrese Gibson – Award-winning singer and actor.

Tyson

Meaning: Firebrand (A person very passionate about a cause)
Origin: Old French
Influential Person: Tyson Gay – American sprinter.

Mike Tyson – Former heavyweight boxing champion of the world.

U

Usain

Meaning: Likely derived from Husain meaning beautiful
Origin: Arabic
Influential Person: Usain Bolt – 8 times Olympic gold medalist and considered the greatest sprinter of all time.

Usher

Meaning: Usher
Origin: English
Influential Person: Usher Raymond – Grammy award-winning singer and songwriter.

V

Victor

Meaning: Winner, conqueror
Origin: Latin
Influential Person: Victor Wooten – Grammy award-winning American bassist.

Virgil

Meaning: Staff bearer
Origin: Latin
Influential Person: Virgil Abloh – American fashion designer and founder of Off White.

W

Walter

Meaning: Commander of the army
Origin: German
Influential Person: Walter Payton – American football player, widely regarded as one of the greatest of all time.

Wesley

Meaning: Western meadow
Origin: English
Influential Person: Wesley Snipes – Award-winning actor and black belt martial artist.

Will

Meaning: Protector
Origin: English
Influential Person: Will Smith – Award-winning actor, rapper, and film producer.

William

Meaning: Determined, resolute protector
Origin: English
Influential Person: William Wells Brown – Activist and author. He was the first African American to have a novel published.

Wyclef

Meaning: Dweller at the white cliff
Origin: English
Influential Person: Wyclef Jean – Grammy award-winning Haitian rapper.

Wylie

Meaning: Clever, crafty
Origin: Old English
Influential Person: Wylie (Richard Kylea Cowie Jr.) – British rapper, songwriter, and record producer. "The Godfather of Grime", he was a key figure in the creation of Grime.

POPULAR

"Remember that a person's name is to that person the sweetest and most important sound in any language."

Boy ♂

A

Ace
Meaning: Unity
Origin: Latin

Adonis
Meaning: Lord
Origin: Greek

Afi
Meaning: Fire
Origin: Polynesian

Africa
Meaning: From Africa
Origin: African

Akeem
Meaning: Intelligent, wise
Origin: Arabic

Akio
Meaning: Bright, clear
Origin: Japanese

Alexander
Meaning: Defender of men
Origin: Greek

Alexis
Meaning: Helper, defender
Origin: Greek

Ali
Meaning: High, elevated, champion
Origin: Arabic

Ameer
Meaning: Prince, chief
Origin: Arabic

Andreas
Meaning: Manly
Origin: Greek

Antoine
Meaning: Derived from Anton meaning priceless
Origin: Latin

Aren
Meaning: Eagle, ruler, peace
Origin: German

Atlas
Meaning: Enduring
Origin: Greek

Azariah
Meaning: Helped by God
Origin: Unknown

B

Bali
Meaning: Strength
Origin: Unknown

Barack
Meaning: Blessing
Origin: African

Ben/Benjamin
Meaning: Son of my right hand
Origin: Hebrew

Blair
Meaning: Field, plain
Origin: Scottish

Blake
Meaning: Dark
Origin: English

C

Cairo
Meaning: Victorious
Origin: Arabic

Cameron
Meaning: Crooked nose
Origin: Scottish

Carey
Meaning: From the fort
Origin: irish

Carter
Meaning: Cart driver
Origin: English

Cartier
Meaning: Cart driver
Origin: French

Casey
Meaning: Vigilant
Origin: Gaelic

Chad
Meaning: Battle warrior
Origin: English

Chai
Meaning: Life
Origin: Hebrew

Christian
Meaning: Follower of Christ
Origin: Hebrew

Cleveland
Meaning: From the cliff
Origin: English

Cole
Meaning: Victorious people
Origin: Greek

Colin
Meaning: Young man
Origin: Gaelic

Corey
Meaning: Hollow
Origin: Irish

Courtney
Meaning: From the court
Origin: English

D

Daniel
Meaning: God is my judge
Origin: Hebrew

Dayo
Meaning: Happiness has come
Origin: African

Delta
Meaning: Born fourth
Origin: Greek

Denali
Meaning: Great one
Origin: Native American

Deon
Meaning: God
Origin: Greek

Dexter
Meaning: One who dyes
Origin: English

Drake
Meaning: Dragon
Origin: English

E

Eli
Meaning: High, elevated
Origin: Hebrew

Elon
Meaning: Oak tree
Origin: Hebrew

Ermias
Meaning: God will uplift
Origin: African

Ethan
Meaning: Firm, strong
Origin: Hebrew

Evan
Meaning: The Lord is gracious
Origin: Welsh

Everest
Meaning: Dweller from the Eure river. Also, the tallest mountain in the world.
Origin: English

Ezekiel
Meaning: God will strengthen
Origin: Hebrew

G

Garvey
Meaning: Rough peace
Origin: Gaelic

Ghana
Meaning: A country in Africa. The word means "warrior king"
Origin: African

H

Hamilton
Meaning: From the mountain town
Origin: Unknown

I

Ilori
Meaning: Special treasure
Origin: African

Ira
Meaning: Watchful one
Origin: Hebrew

Isaac
Meaning: He will laugh
Origin: Hebrew

Isaiah
Meaning: Salvation of God
Origin: Hebrew

Ixia
Meaning: South African flower
Origin: African

J

Jabari
Meaning: Brave one
Origin: Swahili

Jace
Meaning: Healer
Origin: Greek

Jackson
Meaning: Son of Jack
Origin: Unknown

Jacob
Meaning: Supplanter
Origin: Hebrew

Jade
Meaning: Stone of the side
Origin: Spanish

Jaden
Meaning: God has heard
Origin: Hebrew

Jamal
Meaning: Handsome
Origin: Arabic

James
Meaning: Supplanter, replacer
Origin: Hebrew

Jason
Meaning: Healer
Origin: Greek

Jasper
Meaning: Treasurer
Origin: Persian

Jeremiah
Meaning: Appointed by God
Origin: Hebrew

Jerome
Meaning: Sacred name
Origin: Greek

Joe
Meaning: God will give
Origin: Hebrew

Jordan
Meaning: Flowing down
Origin: Hebrew

Joseph
Meaning: God increases
Origin: Hebrew

Joshua
Meaning: The Lord is my salvation
Origin: Hebrew

K

Kai
Meaning: Sea
Origin: Hawaiian

Kaia
Meaning: The sea
Origin: Hawaiian

Kairo
Meaning: Victorious
Origin: Arabic

Kairu
Meaning: Black one
Origin: African

Kalen
Meaning: Strong leader
Origin: Gaelic

Karume
Meaning: Master
Origin: Swahili

Kauri
Meaning: Tree
Origin: Maori

Keanu
Meaning: Cool breeze over the mountains
Origin: Hawaiian

Kellan
Meaning: Slender
Origin: Gaelic

Kemal
Meaning: Perfection
Origin: Turkish

Kenan
Meaning: Possession
Origin: Hebrew

Kendrick
Meaning: Greatest champion, bold ruler
Origin: Welsh

Kenji
Meaning: Intelligent, strong
Origin: Japanese

Kevin
Meaning: Handsome
Origin: Irish

Khari
Meaning: Kingly
Origin: Swahili

Kimoni
Meaning: A great man
Origin: African

Kingsley
Meaning: From The king's meadow
Origin: English

Koa
Meaning: Brave
Origin: Haiwaiian

Kobe
Meaning: God will protect
Origin: Hebrew

Kojo
Meaning: Born on a Monday
Origin: African

Kwame
Meaning: Born on a Saturday
Origin: African

Kwanza
Meaning: Beginning, birth. Also, an annual holiday celebrated by Black people
Origin: African–Swahili

Kyle
Meaning: Narrow
Origin: Scottish

Kyo
Meaning: Apricot
Origin: Unknown

L

Lamar
Meaning: The water, of the sea
Origin: German

Lebron
Meaning: King
Origin: African

Levi
Meaning: Joined
Origin: Hebrew

Lewis
Meaning: Famed warrior
Origin: English

Logan
Meaning: Little hollow
Origin: Scottish

Luca
Meaning: Light
Origin: Latin

Lucas
Meaning: Giver of light
Origin: Latin

M

Maddox
Meaning: Generous
Origin: Welsh

Maia
Meaning: Great
Origin: Latin

Malik
Meaning: King
Origin: Arabic

Marcus
Meaning: Follower of Mars (Roman God of war)
Origin: Latin

Martell
Meaning: Warrior of Mars (Roman God of war)
Origin: German

Marvin
Meaning: Lives by the sea
Origin: Welsh

Mason
Meaning: Stone worker, bricklayer
Origin: English

Mateo
Meaning: Gift from God
Origin: Hebrew

Micah
Meaning: Who is like God?
Origin: Hebrew

Miles
Meaning: Soldier
Origin: Latin

Milo
Meaning: Merciful
Origin: British

Mukisa
Meaning: Good fortune or luck
Origin: Unknown

N

Nate
Meaning: God has given
Origin: Hebrew

Nathaniel
Meaning: Gift of God
Origin: Hebrew

Neo/Neyo
Meaning: Gift
Origin: African/American

Nile/Nyle
Meaning: Champion
Origin: Gaelic

Noah
Meaning: Rest, comfort
Origin: Hebrew

Noel
Meaning: Born on Christmas
Origin: French

Nyall
Meaning: Champion
Origin: Unknown

O

Ocean
Meaning: Sea
Origin: Greek

Odin
Meaning: Frenzy, eager
Origin: Norse

Oliver
Meaning: Olive tree
Origin: French

Omari
Meaning: Flourishing
Origin: Arabic

Orion
Meaning: Rising in the sky
Origin: Greek

Oscar
Meaning: Spear of the gods
Origin: Scandinavian

Otis
Meaning: Rich, wealth, prosperous
Origin: English

Ozias
Meaning: Strength from the Lord
Origin: Greek

P

Phoenix
Meaning: Dark red
Origin: Greek

Prince
Meaning: Leader
Origin: Latin

Psalm
Meaning: Song
Origin: Greek

Q

Quentin
Meaning: The fifth one
Origin: Latin

R

Raden
Meaning: God of thunder
Origin: Japanese

Raine
Meaning: Mighty
Origin: Scandinavian

Rayne
Meaning: Song
Origin: Scandinavian

Remi
Meaning: Oarsman
Origin: French

Ren
Meaning: Lotus
Origin: Japanese

Reuben
Meaning: Behold a son
Origin: Hebrew

Revel
Meaning: Rejoice
Origin: English

Riley
Meaning: Courageous
Origin: British

Rio
Meaning: River
Origin: Spanish

Roman
Meaning: Citizen of Rome
Origin: Latin

Ruby
Meaning: A deep red precious stone
Origin: Latin

S

Saint
Meaning: Holy person
Origin: American

Sean
Meaning: God is gracious
Origin: Irish

Shakir
Meaning: Thankful
Origin: Arabic

Shawn/Sean
Meaning: God is gracious
Origin: Irish

Shiloh
Meaning: Tranquil
Origin: Hebrew

Stormy
Meaning: Impetuous nature
Origin: American

T

Terrell
Meaning: To pull
Origin: French

Theo
Meaning: God
Origin: Greek

Tion
Meaning: Steadfast, firm
Origin: American

Trayvon
Meaning: Brave one
Origin: American

Tristan
Meaning: Sad
Origin: Celtic

Tyler
Meaning: Maker of tiles
Origin: English

Tyson

Meaning: Firebrand (a person very passionate about a cause)
Origin: Old French

U

Usain

Meaning: Likely derived from Husain meaning beautiful
Origin: Arabic

V

Valentino

Meaning: Strong
Origin: Italian

W

Wade

Meaning: To go
Origin: English

Will

Meaning: Protector
Origin: English

Winter

Meaning: Cold season
Origin: American

Y

Yao

Meaning: Born on Thursday
Origin: African–Ghana

Z

Zariah
Meaning: Radiance
Origin: Arabic

Zayne
Meaning: God is gracious
Origin: Hebrew

Zen
Meaning: Meditation
Origin: Japanese

Zeren
Meaning: Golden
Origin: Arabic

Zion
Meaning: Highest place
Origin: Hebrew

Zyan
Meaning: Little king
Origin: English

ARABIC

"And when the heart loves something, the eyes see it as Paradise."

Boy ♂

A

Abdalla
Meaning: Servant of God
Origin: Arabic

Abdullah
Meaning: Servant of God
Origin: Arabic

Abidin
Meaning: Worshippers, adorers
Origin: Arabic

Adlan
Meaning: Fair, just
Origin: Arabic

Adnan
Meaning: Settler
Origin: Arabic

Afeez
Meaning: A path to paradise
Origin: Arabic

Ahamad
Meaning: Highly praised
Origin: Arabic

Ahmed
Meaning: Highly praised
Origin: Arabic

Akeem
Meaning: Intelligent, wise
Origin: Arabic

Akhyar
Meaning: Best, excellent
Origin: Arabic

Akil
Meaning: Intelligent
Origin: Arabic

Akram
Meaning: Most generous
Origin: Arabic

Alem
Meaning: Wise man, highly qualified
Origin: Arabic

Alimayu
Meaning: In God's honor
Origin: African - Ethiopia

Aman
Meaning: Security, peace
Origin: Arabic

Amana
Meaning: Security, peace
Origin: Arabic

Amani
Meaning: Wishes
Origin: Arabic

Amar
Meaning: Long life, immortal
Origin: Arabic

Ameer
Meaning: Prince, chief
Origin: Arabic

Amin
Meaning: Honest, faithful, trustworthy
Origin: Arabic

Amiri
Meaning: Prince
Origin: Arabic

Ara
Meaning: King, brings rain
Origin: Arabic

Asim
Meaning: Protector
Origin: Arabic

Asma
Meaning: High status
Origin: Arabic

Assad
Meaning: Lion
Origin: Arabic

Aswad
Meaning: Black
Origin: Arabic

Azeem
Meaning: Protector
Origin: Arabic

B

Barack
Meaning: Blessing
Origin: Arabic

Baraka
Meaning: Blessing
Origin: Arabic

Basim
Meaning: Smiling
Origin: Arabic

Basit
Meaning: Creator
Origin: Arabic

C

Cairo
Meaning: Victorious
Origin: Arabic

Carim
Meaning: Generous
Origin: Arabic

Chafik
Meaning: Sympathizing
Origin: Arabic

Coman
Meaning: Noble
Origin: Arabic

D

Daiyan
Meaning: A mighty ruler, judge
Origin: Arabic

Daniel
Meaning: God is my judge
Origin: Hebrew

Darim
Meaning: One who takes short steps
Origin: Arabic

Djamel
Meaning: Beauty
Origin: Arabic

E

Eman
Meaning: Belief, faith
Origin: Arabic

Emran
Meaning: Progress, achievement
Origin: Arabic

F

Fadil
Meaning: Generous
Origin: Arabic

Fahim
Meaning: Intelligent, scholar
Origin: Arabic

Fardeen
Meaning: One who has triple strength
Origin: Arabic

Farouk
Meaning: The one who knows right from wrong
Origin: Arabic

Fayad
Meaning: Benefit, advantage, welfare
Origin: Arabic

G

Ghasan
Meaning: Youth, prime of Life
Origin: Arabic

Ghiyas
Meaning: One who asks for help
Origin: Arabic

Givon
Meaning: Hill, high place
Origin: Arabic

H

Habib
Meaning: Loved one
Origin: Arabic

Habibullah
Meaning: Beloved of God
Origin: Arabic

Hafiz
Meaning: Protector
Origin: Arabic

Hakeem
Meaning: Wise
Origin: Arabic

Hamza
Meaning: Lion
Origin: Arabic

Hassan
Meaning: Benefactor
Origin: Arabic

Helal
Meaning: First moon
Origin: Arabic

Husani
Meaning: Handsome
Origin: Arabic

I

Ibrahim
Meaning: Father of many
Origin: Arabic

Ifran
Meaning: One with an Identity
Origin: Arabic

Iman
Meaning: Faith
Origin: Arabic

Iyaaz
Meaning: Generous, bountiful
Origin: Arabic

J

Jafari
Meaning: Stream, creek
Origin: Arabic

Jalaal
Meaning: Grandeur, glory of the faith
Origin: Arabic

Jamaal
Meaning: Handsome, grace
Origin: Arabic

Jamal
Meaning: Handsome
Origin: Arabic

Javan
Meaning: Youth
Origin: Arabic

Jawhar
Meaning: Jewel
Origin: Arabic

Jericho
Meaning: City of moons
Origin: Arabic

Jibril/Jubril
Meaning: Angel
Origin: Arabic

Jimar
Meaning: Handsome
Origin: Arabic

K

Kadeem
Meaning: Servant
Origin: Arabic

Kahlil
Meaning: Friend
Origin: Arabic

Kairo
Meaning: Victorious
Origin: Arabic

Kamaal
Meaning: Perfection
Origin: Arabic

Kamar
Meaning: Moon
Origin: Arabic

Karam
Meaning: Generosity, bounty
Origin: Arabic

Karim
Meaning: Generous
Origin: Arabic

Kasim
Meaning: One who divides goods
Origin: Arabic

Kayden
Meaning: Companion
Origin: Arabic

Khaalid
Meaning: Immortal
Origin: Arabic

Khalan
Meaning: A strong warrior
Origin: Arabic

Khalid
Meaning: Eternal
Origin: Arabic

L

Lateef
Meaning: Gentle, kind
Origin: Arabic

Latif
Meaning: Gentle, kind
Origin: Arabic

M

Maanan
Meaning: Very Generous, bountiful
Origin: Arabic

Malik
Meaning: King
Origin: Arabic

Manal
Meaning: Attainment
Origin: Arabic

Mizan
Meaning: Balance
Origin: Arabic

Muhammad
Meaning: Praiseworthy
Origin: Arabic

N

Nadim
Meaning: Companion, friend
Origin: Arabic

Nadir
Meaning: Rare, scarce
Origin: Arabic

Nassor
Meaning: Supporter
Origin: Arabic

O

Omar
Meaning: Flourishing
Origin: Arabic

Omari
Meaning: Flourishing
Origin: Arabic

Omarion
Meaning: Flourishing
Origin: Arabic

P

Pason
Meaning: Uprising
Origin: Arabic

Pelabo
Meaning: Lightning
Origin: Arabic

Phineas
Meaning: Nubian
Origin: Hebrew

Q

Qabir
Meaning: Very good
Origin: Arabic

Qamar
Meaning: Moon
Origin: Arabic

Qani
Meaning: Satisfied, content
Origin: Arabic

Qaseem
Meaning: Divides, share
Origin: Arabic

Qasit
Meaning: Just, fair
Origin: Arabic

Quasim
Meaning: Just, fair
Origin: Arabic

R

Radd
Meaning: Advisor, counselor
Origin: Arabic

Rashad
Meaning: Good guidance, rightly guided
Origin: Arabic

Rasheed
Meaning: Rightly guided
Origin: Arabic

S

Sabah
Meaning: Morning
Origin: Arabic

Sabir
Meaning: Patient
Origin: Arabic

Saleem
Meaning: Safe
Origin: Arabic

Salim
Meaning: Safe
Origin: Arabic

Sami
Meaning: High (status)
Origin: Arabic

Shakir
Meaning: Thankful
Origin: Arabic

Shakur
Meaning: Thankful
Origin: Arabic

Shaquille
Meaning: Handsome
Origin: Arabic

Sheik
Meaning: Leader, chief
Origin: Arabic

Sultan
Meaning: King
Origin: Arabic

T

Tabari
Meaning: He remembers (like God remembers)
Origin: Arabic

Tahir
Meaning: Pure
Origin: Arabic

Taj
Meaning: Crown
Origin: Arabic

Talum
Meaning: Be sympathetic
Origin: Arabic

Tyrique
Meaning: Saver of the people
Origin: Arabic

U

Ulema

Meaning: Intelligent one
Origin: Arabic

Umar

Meaning: Long life
Origin: Arabic

Umran

Meaning: Prosperity
Origin: Arabic

Usain

Meaning: Likely derived from Husain meaning beautiful
Origin: Arabic

Uzair

Meaning: Helper, strength
Origin: Arabic

V

Vakar

Meaning: Respect, dignity
Origin: Arabic

Vashim

Meaning: Handsome
Origin: Arabic

Vasim

Meaning: Graceful and good-looking
Origin: Arabic

W

Waasif

Meaning: Describing, man of qualities
Origin: Arabic

Waasiq

Meaning: Confident, certain
Origin: Arabic

Wahid

Meaning: Unique
Origin: Arabic

Wali

Meaning: Friend, Lord, governor
Origin: Arabic

X

Xavier
Meaning: Bright, splendid
Origin: Arabic

Xobeen
Meaning: Spear
Origin: Arabic

Y

Yahya
Meaning: Given by God
Origin: Arabic

Yasir
Meaning: Rich
Origin: Arabic

Yusef
Meaning: God will increase
Origin: Arabic

Z

Zahair
Meaning: Helper, supporter
Origin: Arabic

Zahar/Zahir
Meaning: Shine, sparkle, bloom, flourishing
Origin: Arabic

Zahur
Meaning: Eminent
Origin: Arabic

Zaid
Meaning: Abundance, increase
Origin: Arabic

Zain
Meaning: Grace, beauty
Origin: Arabic

Zeeshan
Meaning: Magnificent
Origin: Arabic

Zeren
Meaning: Golden
Origin: Arabic

Zoran
Meaning: Derived from Zora meaning dawn
Origin: Arabic

AFRICAN AMERICAN

"Children are the reward of life."–African Proverb

Boy ♂

A

Antonne
Meaning: Priceless
Origin: Latin

C

Camara
Meaning: Teacher
Origin: African

Charis
Meaning: Grace, kindness
Origin: Greek

Clevon
Meaning: From the cliff
Origin: English

D

Daevon
Meaning: Derived from Davon meaning beloved
Origin: Hebrew

Dajuan
Meaning: God is gracious
Origin: African American

Damany
Meaning: Of bright tomorrow
Origin: African American

Damarion
Meaning: Young bull
Origin: Greek/American

Damon
Meaning: To tame
Origin: Greek

Dandrae
Meaning: Strong, brave, courageous
Origin: Greek

Dangelo
Meaning: From the angel
Origin: Italian

Davion
Meaning: Beloved
Origin: American

Daymond
Meaning: Bright
Origin: English

Deaengelo
Meaning: Of the angels
Origin: Italian

Deandrae
Meaning: Warrior, brave man
Origin: American

Deion
Meaning: God
Origin: African American

Deiondre
Meaning: Valley
Origin: American

Deontay
Meaning: Derived from Deon meaning belongs to God
Origin: Greek

Desean
Meaning: God is gracious
Origin: African American

Deshane
Meaning: Derived from Shaun meaning God is merciful
Origin: American

Deshawn
Meaning: God is gracious
Origin: American

Dijon
Meaning: God is gracious
Origin: Hebrew

Dontrell
Meaning: Lasting, enduring
Origin: American

E

Emiel
Meaning: Rival
Origin: Latin

H

Huxley
Meaning: Hugh's meadow
Origin: English

J

Jaheim
Meaning: Raised up
Origin: Hebrew

Jamaa
Meaning: Supplanter
Origin: Hebrew

Jarell
Meaning: Ruler with the spear
Origin: English

Jaumar
Meaning: Handsome man
Origin: Jamaican

Jawara
Meaning: Lover of peace
Origin: African

Jemarcus
Meaning: From the God Mars
Origin: African American

Jenae
Meaning: God has answered
Origin: Unknown

Jevonte
Meaning: Son of Japheth
Origin: African American

Jimarcus
Meaning: Of Mars, warrior
Origin: Jamaican

Judean
Meaning: Loyal to the king of Judea
Origin: Jamaican

K

Keenan
Meaning: Ancient
Origin: Irish

Kendis
Meaning: Pure
Origin: African American

Keshawn
Meaning: God is gracious
Origin: American

Kobe
Meaning: God will protect
Origin: Hebrew

Kyrone
Meaning: Land of Owen
Origin: American

L

Lasean
Meaning: God is gracious
Origin: American

Lashawn
Meaning: God is gracious
Origin: Hebrew

Lavaughn
Meaning: Little
Origin: American

Lemarcus
Meaning: From the God Mars
Origin: American

M

Makalani
Meaning: Clerk
Origin: African

Mansa
Meaning: Conqueror, king, king of kings
Origin: African

Marquis
Meaning: Nobleman
Origin: French

Mashawn
Meaning: God is gracious
Origin: African American

N

Nashawn
Meaning: God is gracious
Origin: African American

Neo/Neyo
Meaning: Gift
Origin: African/American

O

Omari
Meaning: Flourishing
Origin: Arabic

Omarion
Meaning: Flourishing
Origin: Arabic

P

Perry
Meaning: Traveler, wanderer
Origin: American

Q

Quashawn
Meaning: A tenacious man, tenacious
Origin: African American

R

Rachard
Meaning: Righteous
Origin: Jamaican

Rachiim
Meaning: Seed of rulership
Origin: African American

Raimy
Meaning: Celebration
Origin: American

Ramell
Meaning: Son
Origin: Jamaican

Rashad
Meaning: Good guidance, rightly guided
Origin: Arabic

Rasheed
Meaning: Rightly guided
Origin: Arabic

Rashon
Meaning: God is gracious
Origin: American

Reggis
Meaning: Ruler with counsel
Origin: American

Reshay
Meaning: A gift
Origin: Jamaican

Ricki
Meaning: Brave ruler
Origin: American

Roshaun
Meaning: Shining light
Origin: Sanskrit

S

Sardis
Meaning: Prince of joy
Origin: Biblical

T

Tavon
Meaning: Nature
Origin: Scottish

Taye
Meaning: He has been seen
Origin: African

Teneil
Meaning: Champion
Origin: American

Tiger
Meaning: Powerful cat
Origin: American

Tinashe
Meaning: God is with us
Origin: African

Tion
Meaning: Steadfast, firm
Origin: American

Trayvon
Meaning: Brave one
Origin: American

Tremaine
Meaning: From a town built by stone
Origin: Celtic

Tupac
Meaning: Royal
Origin: American

Tyler
Meaning: Maker of tiles
Origin: English

V

Vashon
Meaning: God Is gracious, merciful
Origin: American

W

Wakili
Meaning: Lawyer, representative
Origin: African

Wali
Meaning: Friend, Lord, governor
Origin: Arabic

X

Xayvion
Meaning: The new house
Origin: African American

Xoese
Meaning: Believe, faith
Origin: African

Z

Zakari
Meaning: The Lord recalled
Origin: Hebrew

Zambga
Meaning: First born
Origin: African American

Zeshawn
Meaning: God is gracious, merciful
Origin: African American

MODERN

"Words have meanings. Names have power."

Boy ♂

A

Adjo
Meaning: Righteous
Origin: African

Ahanti
Meaning: Eternal, indestructible, warlike
Origin: Hindi

Aiyetoro
Meaning: Peace on Earth
Origin: African

Aldrin
Meaning: Old
Origin: Unknown

Alessio
Meaning: Defender
Origin: Old German

Alexis
Meaning: Helper, defender
Origin: Greek

Alonzo
Meaning: Ready
Origin: Spanish

Alvin
Meaning: Noble friend
Origin: English

Alwyn
Meaning: Wise friend
Origin: English

Alyssa
Meaning: Noble
Origin: English

Ame
Meaning: Beloved
Origin: Latin

Anando
Meaning: Bliss
Origin: Sanskrit

Andreas
Meaning: Manly
Origin: Greek

Andres
Meaning: Manly
Origin: Spanish

Andrin
Meaning: Ruler of the home
Origin: Old German

Aoko
Meaning: Blue child
Origin: Japanese

Apollo
Meaning: Destroyer
Origin: Greek

Ara
Meaning: King, brings rain
Origin: Arabic

Archer
Meaning: Bowman. Also refers to the Sagittarius constellation
Origin: English

Ario
Meaning: Belligerent
Origin: Italian

Armani
Meaning: Warrior
Origin: Italian

Arris
Meaning: Best
Origin: Latin

Ashanti
Meaning: The name of a tribe in Ghana
Origin: African

Aspen
Meaning: Aspen tree
Origin: Old English

Aston
Meaning: From the East town
Origin: English

Avery
Meaning: Ruler of the elves, wise
Origin: French

Ayden
Meaning: Little fire
Origin: Irish

B

Bailey
Meaning: Agent of the law
Origin: Old English

Baron
Meaning: Noble person
Origin: English

Bash
Meaning: Chief commander
Origin: Turkish

Basil
Meaning: Kingly
Origin: Greek

Beau
Meaning: Beautiful
Origin: French

Benton
Meaning: Settlement near the moor
Origin: English

Berton
Meaning: Bright settlement
Origin: German

Boston
Meaning: By the woods
Origin: Unknown

Bradley
Meaning: Broad meadow
Origin: English

Bron
Meaning: Brown, dark
Origin: French

Brooklyn
Meaning: Beautiful brook
Origin: Unknown

Bryson
Meaning: Son of nobleman
Origin: English

Byron
Meaning: Cow barn
Origin: Old English

C

Calbert
Meaning: Cowherd, cowboy
Origin: British

Calian
Meaning: Warrior of life
Origin: Native American

Cameron
Meaning: Crooked nose
Origin: Scottish

Carey
Meaning: From the fort
Origin: Irish

Carlos
Meaning: Free man
Origin: Spanish

Carlton
Meaning: From the town of the free men
Origin: Unknown

Carnell
Meaning: Defender of the castle
Origin: English

Carson
Meaning: Son of marsh dwellers
Origin: Unknown

Cartier
Meaning: Cart driver
Origin: French

Cary
Meaning: Pure
Origin: English

Caspar
Meaning: Keeper of the treasure
Origin: Persian

Cassius
Meaning: Vain
Origin: Latin

Cavelle
Meaning: Small and active
Origin: Unknown

Cavin
Meaning: Beautiful at birth
Origin: German

Chafik
Meaning: Sympathizing
Origin: Arabic

Chafulumisa
Meaning: Fast
Origin: African-Egypt

Chance
Meaning: Fortune
Origin: English

Chase
Meaning: Huntsman
Origin: French

Chester
Meaning: A fortress, camp
Origin: Latin

Chicago
Meaning: Onion
Origin: Unknown

Ciaran
Meaning: Dark Haired
Origin: Irish

Clifton
Meaning: Town by the cliff
Origin: English

Cody
Meaning: Cushion, pillow
Origin: English

Colt
Meaning: Young horse
Origin: British

Cordell
Meaning: A rope maker
Origin: English

Cornelius
Meaning: Horn
Origin: English

Cornell
Meaning: Derived from Cornelius meaning horn
Origin: French

Cosmo
Meaning: Harmony, order
Origin: Italian

Cruiz
Meaning: Cross
Origin: Unknown

Cruz
Meaning: Cross
Origin: Spanish

Cuba
Meaning: Where fertile land is abundant
Origin: Unknown

Cyan
Meaning: Light blue-green
Origin: American

D

Dace
Meaning: Of nobility
Origin: French

Dallas
Meaning: The meadow dwelling
Origin: Unknown

Damarion
Meaning: Young bull
Origin: Greek

Dameon
Meaning: To tame
Origin: Greek

Dante
Meaning: Lasting
Origin: Italian

Darnell
Meaning: Hidden
Origin: Old English

Dasante
Meaning: Real
Origin: African American

Dayton
Meaning: Day town, light town
Origin: English

Deaengelo
Meaning: Of the angels
Origin: Italian

Dell
Meaning: Small valley
Origin: English

Demont
Meaning: Mountain
Origin: French

Denver
Meaning: Green valley
Origin: Unknown

Deron
Meaning: Belongs to God
Origin: Armenian

Deshawn
Meaning: God is gracious
Origin: American

Devon
Meaning: From Devonshire
Origin: English

Dewayne
Meaning: Dark complexioned
Origin: Irish

Dexter
Meaning: One who dyes
Origin: English

Dion
Meaning: Divine
Origin: Greek

Dior
Meaning: Golden
Origin: French

Djamel
Meaning: Beauty
Origin: Arabic

Donavon
Meaning: Dark
Origin: Unknown

Donell
Meaning: World ruler
Origin: Scottish

Donovan
Meaning: Dark haired
Origin: Irish

Dontrell
Meaning: Lasting, enduring
Origin: American

Duante
Meaning: Dark
Origin: Irish

Dune
Meaning: Brown skinned soldier
Origin: Scottish

Duron
Meaning: Strong
Origin: French

Duval
Meaning: Of the valley
Origin: French

E

Eaton
Meaning: Island settlement
Origin: English

Eddison
Meaning: Son of Edward
Origin: English

Eddy
Meaning: Wealthy protector
Origin: English

Ede
Meaning: Strife for wealth
Origin: English

Eden
Meaning: Place of pleasure
Origin: Hebrew

Elois
Meaning: Famous warrior
Origin: German

Elvan
Meaning: Colorful
Origin: Turkish

Emiel
Meaning: Rival
Origin: Latin

Enzo
Meaning: Home ruler
Origin: Italian

Eric
Meaning: Eternal ruler
Origin: Norse

Ervin
Meaning: Beautiful
Origin: Scottish

Esaia
Meaning: God saves
Origin: Hebrew

Ethan
Meaning: Firm, strong
Origin: Hebrew

F

Falon
Meaning: In charge
Origin: Irish

Farrell
Meaning: Hero, man of courage
Origin: Irish

Ferric
Meaning: Iron
Origin: Latin

Fifi
Meaning: Jehovah increases
Origin: French

Florian
Meaning: Flowerin, flourishing
Origin: Latin

Flynn
Meaning: Son of the red-haired one
Origin: Irish

Fremont
Meaning: Guardian of freedom, free man
Origin: German

G

Garvey
Meaning: Rough peace
Origin: Gaelic

Gene
Meaning: Born Lucky
Origin: Greek

Ghana
Meaning: A country in Africa. The word means "warrior king"
Origin: African

Glover
Meaning: One who makes gloves
Origin: English

H

Hakeem
Meaning: Wise
Origin: Arabic

Hari
Meaning: Lion
Origin: Sanskrit

Harley
Meaning: The long field
Origin: British

Harper
Meaning: Harp player
Origin: English

Harry
Meaning: Home ruler
Origin: Unknown

Harvey
Meaning: Battle worthy
Origin: Unknown

Hayden
Meaning: Hay valley
Origin: English

Hector
Meaning: To restrain
Origin: Greek

Hunter
Meaning: One who hunts
Origin: English

Huxley
Meaning: Hugh's meadow
Origin: English

I

Idris
Meaning: Fiery leader
Origin: Arabic

Israel
Meaning: May God prevail
Origin: Unknown

J

Jace
Meaning: Healer
Origin: Greek

Jafari
Meaning: Stream, creek
Origin: Arabic

Jaheim
Meaning: Raised up
Origin: Hebrew

Jahim
Meaning: Dignity
Origin: Swahili

Jai
Meaning: Champion
Origin: Sanskrit

Jalen
Meaning: Tranquil
Origin: American

Jamaar
Meaning: Handsome, grace
Origin: American

Jameson
Meaning: Son of James
Origin: British

Janus
Meaning: Gateway
Origin: Latin

Jarek
Meaning: Spring
Origin: Slavic

Jarell
Meaning: Ruler with the spear
Origin: English

Jarius
Meaning: To stand out and shine
Origin: Greek

Jarvis
Meaning: Spear man
Origin: English

Jaumar
Meaning: Handsome man
Origin: Jamaican

Jaxon
Meaning: Son of Jack
Origin: English

Jay
Meaning: Blue crested bird
Origin: Latin

Jaydene
Meaning: Thankful
Origin:

Jazz
Meaning: Derived from Jasmine meaning gift from God
Origin: Persian

Jemarcus
Meaning: From the Roman God Mars
Origin: African American

Jenae
Meaning: God has answered
Origin: Unknown

Jenue
Meaning: From Jenue in Nigeria
Origin: African

Jermaine
Meaning: Brother
Origin: Latin

Jerome
Meaning: Sacred name
Origin: Greek

Jerrett
Meaning: Strength of the spear, brave
Origin: German

Jeso
Meaning: God is my salvation
Origin: Basotho

Jet
Meaning: Black stone
Origin: British

Jojo
Meaning: God raises
Origin: Hebrew

Jonah
Meaning: Dove
Origin: Unknown

Jorell
Meaning: Father
Origin: American

Jovan
Meaning: God is gracious
Origin: Slavic

Judge
Meaning: Decision maker
Origin: English

Jules
Meaning: Youthful
Origin: French

Justin
Meaning: Fair, righteous
Origin: Latin

K

Kai
Meaning: Sea
Origin: Hawaiian

Kaleb
Meaning: Whole-hearted
Origin: Hebrew

Karma
Meaning: Fate, destiny
Origin: Sanskrit

Kato
Meaning: All-knowing
Origin: Latin

Kaven
Meaning: Handsome
Origin: Irish

Kaya
Meaning: Rock
Origin: Turkish

Kaylen
Meaning: Keeper of the keys
Origin: English

Kayne
Meaning: Little battle
Origin: Gaelic

Kayson
Meaning: Healer
Origin: Greek

Keanne
Meaning: Sharp
Origin: Celtic

Kei
Meaning: Joyful
Origin: Japanese

Kele
Meaning: Sparrow
Origin: Native American

Kellan
Meaning: Slender
Origin: Gaelic

Kelvin
Meaning: Friend of ships
Origin: English

Kemal
Meaning: Perfection
Origin: Turkish

Kendal
Meaning: Valley of the river Kent
Origin: English

Kendrick
Meaning: Greatest champion, bold ruler
Origin: Welsh

Kenton
Meaning: The royal settlement
Origin: English

Keon
Meaning: God is gracious
Origin: Irish

Keshawn
Meaning: God is gracious
Origin: American

Keyon
Meaning: God is gracious
Origin: Irish

Khalon
Meaning: Strong warrior
Origin: American

Khama
Meaning: Embodiment of forgiveness
Origin: Indian

Kian
Meaning: God is gracious
Origin: Irish

Kiano
Meaning: The wizard tools
Origin: African

Kimbel
Meaning: War leader
Origin: Celtic

Kingston
Meaning: King's settlement
Origin: British

Kinsley
Meaning: King's meadow
Origin: British

Kione
Meaning: Someone who comes from nowhere
Origin: African

Kobe
Meaning: God will protect
Origin: Hebrew

Kordell
Meaning: Cord maker
Origin: English

Kyan
Meaning: Ancient
Origin: Irish

Kylan
Meaning: Straight
Origin: Gaelic

Kyrie
Meaning: Lord
Origin: Greek

Kyrone
Meaning: Land of Owen
Origin: American

L

Lado
Meaning: Great or famous ruler
Origin: Georgian

Laken
Meaning: From the lake
Origin: English

Lamar
Meaning: The water, of the sea
Origin: German

Lamont
Meaning: Law man
Origin: Norse

Lamu
Meaning: Land
Origin: Unknown

Landon
Meaning: From the long hill
Origin: English

Lareina
Meaning: The queen
Origin: Spanish

Lashawn
Meaning: God is gracious
Origin: Hebrew

Lathan
Meaning: God has given
Origin: English

Latrell
Meaning: One who is noble and eager
Origin: American

Lavaughn
Meaning: Little
Origin: American

Lawrence
Meaning: Man from Laurentum
Origin: Latin

Legend
Meaning: Story, myth
Origin: English

Leighton
Meaning: Meadow settlement
Origin: British

Lenka
Meaning: Torch of light
Origin: Greek

Leo
Meaning: Lion
Origin: Latin

Leron
Meaning: The circle
Origin: French

Levon
Meaning: Lion
Origin: Armenian

Lewis
Meaning: Famed warrior
Origin: English

Lincoln
Meaning: From the lake settlement
Origin: English

Linden
Meaning: Made from linwood, lime tree
Origin: English

Logan
Meaning: Little hollow
Origin: Scottish

London
Meaning: From the great river
Origin: Latin

Louis
Meaning: Famous warrior
Origin: German

Lovell
Meaning: Wolf
Origin: French

Lucas
Meaning: Giver of light
Origin: Latin

Lucius
Meaning: Light
Origin: Latin

Lux
Meaning: Light
Origin: Latin

Lynx
Meaning: Brightness
Origin: Greek

Lyron
Meaning: My song
Origin: Hebrew

M

Madison
Meaning: Gift from God
Origin: English

Magic
Meaning: Full of wonder
Origin: American

Malakai
Meaning: My messenger
Origin: Unknown

Maleko
Meaning: Warrior
Origin: Hawaiian

Mario
Meaning: Warlike
Origin: Latin

Maron
Meaning: Little master
Origin: Greek

Marques
Meaning: Nobleman
Origin: French

Marquis
Meaning: Nobleman
Origin: French

Martell
Meaning: Warrior of Mars (Roman God of War)
Origin: German

Mashawn
Meaning: God is gracious
Origin: African American

Mason
Meaning: Stone Worker, bricklayer
Origin: English

Mato
Meaning: Bear
Origin: Native American

Maverick
Meaning: Independent, non-conforming
Origin: English

Meldon
Meaning: From the hillside mill
Origin: British

Melea
Meaning: Complete, full
Origin: Hebrew

Merritt
Meaning: Boundary gate
Origin: English

Moana
Meaning: Ocean, sea
Origin: Hawaiian

Montell
Meaning: My ruler
Origin: French

Morocco
Meaning: A country in Africa
Origin: African

Myles
Meaning: Soldier
Origin: Latin

N

Nait
Meaning: Little gift
Origin: Hebrew

Napoleon
Meaning: Lion of Naples
Origin: Italian

Nero
Meaning: Strong
Origin: Latin

Neron
Meaning: Strong
Origin: Spanish

Nevin
Meaning: Holy, sacred
Origin: Latin

Nile
Meaning: Champion. Also the longest river in Africa.
Origin: Irish

Nile/Nyle
Meaning: Champion
Origin: Gaelic

O

Odai

Meaning: Possibly derived from Uday meaning rise, ascend, to appear
Origin: Sanskrit

Omar

Meaning: Flourishing
Origin: Arabic

Omarion

Meaning: Flourishing
Origin: Arabic

Oree

Meaning: Light
Origin: Hebrew

Orlando

Meaning: Famous throughout the land
Origin: Unknown

Oscar

Meaning: Spear of the gods
Origin: Scandinavian

Owen

Meaning: Noble, youthful, and well-born
Origin: Celtic

P

Pablo

Meaning: Small
Origin: Spanish

Palmer

Meaning: Pilgrim
Origin: English

Paxton

Meaning: Peace
Origin: Latin

Payne

Meaning: Pagan
Origin: English

Payton

Meaning: Fighting man's estate
Origin: English

Perry

Meaning: Traveler, wanderer
Origin: American

Phineas
Meaning: Nubian
Origin: Hebrew

Pierre
Meaning: Rock
Origin: French

Preston
Meaning: The priest's town
Origin: English

Prince
Meaning: Leader
Origin: Latin

Princeton
Meaning: Princely town
Origin: English

Q

Quentin
Meaning: The fifth one
Origin: Latin

Queran
Meaning: Dark haired one
Origin: Irish

Quesnel
Meaning: From the little oak tree
Origin: French

Quetzal
Meaning: Large brilliant tail feather
Origin: American

Quincy
Meaning: Born fifth, fifth
Origin: Latin

Quinn
Meaning: Descendant of Conn
Origin: Irish

R

Raden
Meaning: God of thunder
Origin: Japanese

Raimy
Meaning: Celebration
Origin: American

Rain
Meaning: Rain
Origin: British

Ramell
Meaning: Son
Origin: Jamaican

Ramon
Meaning: Counsel protection
Origin: Spanish/German

Ramone
Meaning: Protecting hands
Origin: Spanish

Randall
Meaning: Wolf shield
Origin: English

Ranger
Meaning: Guardian of the forest
Origin: French

Raphael
Meaning: God has healed
Origin: Hebrew

Raul
Meaning: Wolf counsel
Origin: Spanish/German

Raymond
Meaning: Counsel protection
Origin: English/German

Raynard
Meaning: Strong decision
Origin: German

Reagan
Meaning: Little king
Origin: Irish

Reed
Meaning: Red
Origin: British

Reese
Meaning: Enthusiastic
Origin: Welsh

Reggie
Meaning: Ruler's advisor
Origin: Latin

Reggis
Meaning: Ruler with counsel
Origin: American

Ren
Meaning: Lotus
Origin: Japanese

Revel
Meaning: Rejoice
Origin: English

Rex
Meaning: King
Origin: Latin

Rey
Meaning: King
Origin: Spanish

Reymond
Meaning: Protecting hands
Origin: German

Reymundo/Reimundo
Meaning: Guards wisely
Origin: French

Rion
Meaning: King
Origin: Gaelic

River
Meaning: Stream of water that flows to the sea
Origin: English

Robin
Meaning: Famous, bright
Origin: German

Rocket
Meaning: A jet propelled tube
Origin: English

Rodell
Meaning: Famous ruler
Origin: French

Rodney
Meaning: Island near the clearing
Origin: German

Roman
Meaning: Citizen of Rome
Origin: Latin

Romare
Meaning: Derived from Latin meaning a citizen of Rome
Origin: Latin

Royce
Meaning: Famous, son of king
Origin: English

Ruby
Meaning: A deep red precious stone
Origin: Latin

Russell
Meaning: Little red one
Origin: French

Ryder
Meaning: Horseman, rider
Origin: English

S

Safari
Meaning: Journey
Origin: African

Sage
Meaning: Wise
Origin: Old French

Saint
Meaning: Holy person
Origin: American

Samai
Meaning: Peaceful
Origin: Swahili

Santana
Meaning: Follower of St. Ana
Origin: Spanish

Shai
Meaning: Gift
Origin: Hebrew

Shaka
Meaning: Name given to the chief of the Zulu tribe
Origin: African

Shandon
Meaning: Wise
Origin: Gaelic

Sherwin
Meaning: Swift runner
Origin: English

Shia
Meaning: Praise God
Origin: Hebrew

Shontae
Meaning: Being sung
Origin: English

Sisi
Meaning: Born on Sunday
Origin: African

Sloan
Meaning: Warrior
Origin: Scottish

Stacy
Meaning: Resurrection
Origin: English

Storm
Meaning: Tempest
Origin: British

Sydel/Sidell
Meaning: From the wide valley
Origin: English

T

Taiwo
Meaning: First twin to taste the world
Origin: African

Taj
Meaning: Crown
Origin: Arabic

Takeo
Meaning: Strong as bamboo
Origin: Japanese

Takoda
Meaning: A friend to everyone
Origin: Native American

Tarlo
Meaning: Cub of a bear
Origin: Native American

Tauri
Meaning: Young eagle
Origin: Native American

Taye
Meaning: He has been seen
Origin: African

Terrell
Meaning: To pull
Origin: French

Theodore
Meaning: Gift of God
Origin: Greek

Tiger
Meaning: Powerful cat
Origin: American

Tokala
Meaning: Fox
Origin: Native American

Tokyo
Meaning: Eastern capital
Origin: Unknown

Torin
Meaning: Chief
Origin: Gaelic

Travis
Meaning: To cross
Origin: French

Tremaine
Meaning: From a town built by stone
Origin: Celtic

Trey
Meaning: Three
Origin: English

Troy
Meaning: Foot soldier
Origin: Irish

Tyrel
Meaning: God of Battle
Origin: Irish

Tyrese
Meaning:smooth
Origin: Latin

U

Ulysses
Meaning: Wrathful
Origin: Greek

V

Vale
Meaning: Lives in the valley
Origin: Latin

Valente
Meaning: Valiant
Origin: Portuguese

Valentino
Meaning: Strong
Origin: Italian

Vanya
Meaning: God Is gracious
Origin: Slavic

Vashon
Meaning: God Is gracious, merciful
Origin: American

Veda
Meaning: Knowledge or wisdom
Origin: Sanskrit

Verdell
Meaning: Green
Origin: French

Vincent
Meaning: To conquer
Origin: Latin

Virgil
Meaning: Staff bearer
Origin: Latin

Von
Meaning: Hope
Origin: Norse

W

Wade
Meaning: To go
Origin: English

Wallace
Meaning: Foreigner, stranger
Origin: English

Warren
Meaning: Park keeper
Origin: English

Wayan
Meaning: First son
Origin: Indonesian

Waylon
Meaning: Land by the road
Origin: English

Wayne
Meaning: Wagon builder or driver
Origin: English

Wendell
Meaning: Wanderer
Origin: English

Wesley
Meaning: Western meadow
Origin: English

Wilder
Meaning: Untamed, wild
Origin: English

Wylie
Meaning: Clever, crafty
Origin: Old English

X

Xander
Meaning: Defender of the people
Origin: Greek

Xavier
Meaning: Bright, splendid
Origin: Arabic

Xenon
Meaning: Foreigner, stranger
Origin: Greek

Xerxes
Meaning: Ruler over heroes
Origin: Greek

Xian
Meaning: One who lives alone, elegant
Origin: Chinese

Xion
Meaning: Remembrance
Origin: Japanese

Xochitl
Meaning: Flower
Origin: Aztec

Y

Yonah
Meaning: Dove
Origin: Unknown

Yoshi
Meaning: Good luck, respectful
Origin: Japanese

Yoshiro
Meaning: Happy individual
Origin: Japanese

Yuri
Meaning: Farmer
Origin: Unknown

Yvon
Meaning: Archer
Origin: French

Z

Zacharias
Meaning: The Lord has remembered
Origin: Hebrew

Zachary
Meaning: The Lord has remembered
Origin: Hebrew

Zephan
Meaning: Hidden by God
Origin: Hebrew

Zephyr
Meaning: West wind
Origin: Greek

Zerek
Meaning: Ever powerful ruler
Origin: English

Zeus
Meaning: Sky, shine
Origin: Greek

Zion
Meaning: Highest place
Origin: Hebrew

Zulu
Meaning: Heaven. The Zulu Kingdom was a powerful kingdom in Southern Africa in the 1800s. Today the Zulu people are the largest group in South Africa
Origin: African–South Africa

Zyan

Meaning: Little king
Origin: English

CLASSIC

"A good name will shine forever."

Boy ♂

A

Aaron
Meaning: Exalted
Origin: Hebrew

Adam
Meaning: Son of the red Earth
Origin: Hebrew

Ahmed
Meaning: Highly praised
Origin: Arabic

Alan
Meaning: Handsome
Origin: Celtic

Alex
Meaning: Defender
Origin: Italian

Alexander
Meaning: Defender of men
Origin: Greek

Alton
Meaning: Old town
Origin: English

Andre
Meaning: Manly, brave
Origin: French

Andy
Meaning: Manly
Origin: Greek

Antonne
Meaning: Priceless
Origin: Latin

B

Ben
Meaning: Son
Origin: Hebrew

Ben/Benjamin
Meaning: Son of my right hand
Origin: Hebrew

C

Charles
Meaning: Man, strong
Origin: French

Courtney
Meaning: From the court
Origin: English

Curtis
Meaning: Courteous
Origin: English

D

Daniel
Meaning: God is my judge
Origin: Hebrew

David
Meaning: Beloved
Origin: Hebrew

Dean
Meaning: Valley
Origin: Unknown

Dominic
Meaning: Belonging to the Lord
Origin: Latin

Duane
Meaning: Dark
Origin: Irish

E

Eddie
Meaning: Wealthy guardian
Origin: English

F

Femi
Meaning: Love me
Origin: African

G

George
Meaning: Farmer
Origin: Greek

Gerald
Meaning: Spear ruler
Origin: German

I

Ian

Meaning: God is gracious
Origin: Scottish

J

Jackie

Meaning: Likely derived from the name John meaning God is gracious
Origin: Hebrew

Jacob

Meaning: Supplanter
Origin: Hebrew

Jamal

Meaning: Handsome
Origin: Arabic

James

Meaning: Supplanter, replacer
Origin: Hebrew

Joe

Meaning: God will give
Origin: Hebrew

John

Meaning: God is gracious
Origin: Hebrew

Joseph

Meaning: God increases
Origin: Hebrew

K

Karl

Meaning: Free man
Origin: German

Kofi

Meaning: Born on a Friday
Origin: African

L

Leon
Meaning: Lion
Origin: Greek

M

Malcolm
Meaning: Devotee of Saint Columba
Origin: Gaelic

Martin
Meaning: Servant Of Mars (Roman God Of War)
Origin: Latin

Matthew
Meaning: Gift of God
Origin: Hebrew

O

Ola
Meaning: Wealth
Origin: African–Nigeria

P

Patrick
Meaning: Noble man
Origin: English

Pearl
Meaning: Pearl
Origin: Unknown

R

Richard
Meaning: Brave ruler
Origin: English

Robert
Meaning: Bright fame
Origin: German

Russell
Meaning: Little red one
Origin: French

Ryan
Meaning: Little king
Origin: Irish

S

Samuel
Meaning: God has heard
Origin: Hebrew

Shawn/Sean
Meaning: God is gracious
Origin: Irish

T

Terry
Meaning: Powerful
Origin: German

Tony
Meaning: Priceless one
Origin: Latin

W

William
Meaning: Determined, resolute protector
Origin: English

RELIGIOUS

"Babies are a bit of stardust blown from the hands of God."

Boy ♂

A

Abdalla
Meaning: Servant of God
Origin: Arabic

Abdullah
Meaning: Servant of God
Origin: Arabic

Abidin
Meaning: Worshippers, adorers
Origin: Arabic

Abraham
Meaning: Father of multitudes
Origin: Hebrew

Adam
Meaning: Son of the red Earth
Origin: Hebrew

Adiel
Meaning: Ornament of God
Origin: Hebrew

Ahmed
Meaning: Highly praised
Origin: Arabic

Alimayu
Meaning: In God's honor
Origin: African - Ethopia

Adio
Meaning: He is righteous
Origin: African

Adnan
Meaning: Settler
Origin: Arabic

Adom
Meaning: Help from God
Origin: Hebrew

Adonis
Meaning: Lord
Origin: Greek

Ahamad
Meaning: Highly praised
Origin: Arabic

Ahanti
Meaning: Eternal
Origin: Hindi

Amit
Meaning: Friend
Origin: Hebrew

Amos
Meaning: Carried by God
Origin: Hebrew

Andwele

Meaning: God brings me
Origin: Africa

Anthone

Meaning: Highly praised, priceless one
Origin: Latin

Anthony

Meaning: Worthy of praise
Origin: Latin

Antonio

Meaning: Worthy of praise
Origin: Latin

Arie

Meaning: Lion of God
Origin: Hebrew

B

Barachel

Meaning: Blessed by God
Origin: Hebrew

Bartholomew

Meaning: Son of the furrowed
Origin: Aramaic

Bilgah

Meaning: Cheerful
Origin: Hebrew

C

Carim

Meaning: Generous
Origin: Arabic

Chafik

Meaning: Sympathizing
Origin: Arabic

Chetachi

Meaning: Remember God
Origin: African

Chiamaka

Meaning: God is beautiful
Origin: African

Chiazam

Meaning: Answer from God
Origin: African

Chidubem

Meaning: Guided by God
Origin: African

Chiemeka

Meaning: God has performed great deeds
Origin: African

Chijioke

Meaning: Divinity gives talent
Origin: African

Chika

Meaning: Divinity is the greatest
Origin: African

Chikae

Meaning: God's power
Origin: African American

Chike

Meaning: Power of God
Origin: African

Chikezie

Meaning: Well made by God
Origin: african

Chikwendu

Meaning: May God give you life
Origin: African

Chima

Meaning: God knows
Origin: African

Chimelu

Meaning: Made of God
Origin: African

Chinelo

Meaning: Thoughts of God
Origin: African–Nigeria

Chinyelu

Meaning: God gave
Origin: African–Nigeria

Chioke

Meaning: Gift of God
Origin: African–Nigeria

Chioma

Meaning: God is good, great
Origin: African

Christian

Meaning: Follower of Christ
Origin: Hebrew

Christopher

Meaning: Follower of Christ
Origin: latin

Cyrille

Meaning: Lord
Origin: Unknown

D

Dajuan
Meaning: God is gracious
Origin: African American

Dakarai
Meaning: Rejoice
Origin: African

Damani
Meaning: Tomorrow
Origin: American

Dangelo
Meaning: From the angel
Origin: Italian

Daniel
Meaning: God is my judge
Origin: Hebrew

Dejohn
Meaning: God is gracious
Origin: Hebrew

Deon
Meaning: God
Origin: Greek

Deontay
Meaning: Derived from Deon meaning belongs to God
Origin: Greek

Desean
Meaning: God is gracious
Origin: African American

Deshawn
Meaning: God is gracious
Origin: American

Dijon
Meaning: God is gracious
Origin: Hebrew

Dominique
Meaning: Of the Lord
Origin: Latin

E

Elias
Meaning: The Lord is my God
Origin: Hebrew

Elijah
Meaning: Yahweh is my God
Origin: Hebrew

Eman
Meaning: Belief, faith
Origin: Arabic

Emmanuel
Meaning: God is with us
Origin: Hebrew

Esaia
Meaning: God saves
Origin: Hebrew

Ethan
Meaning: Firm, strong
Origin: Hebrew

Evan
Meaning: The Lord is gracious
Origin: Welsh

Ezekiel
Meaning: God will strengthen
Origin: Hebrew

Ezra
Meaning: Helper
Origin: Hebrew

F

Faddey
Meaning: Gift given by God
Origin: Aramaic

Fayad
Meaning: Benefit, advantage, welfare
Origin: Arabic

Foluke
Meaning: Under God's protection
Origin: African

Fortunatus
Meaning: Fortunate
Origin: Latin

G

Gabe
Meaning: God is my strength
Origin: Hebrew

Gabriel
Meaning: God is my strength
Origin: Hebrew

Gabrio
Meaning: God is my strength
Origin: Hebrew

H

Habibullah
Meaning: Beloved of God
Origin: Arabic

Hafiz
Meaning: Protector
Origin: Arabic

Haskell
Meaning: God's helmet
Origin: Norse

Heman
Meaning: Faithful
Origin: Hebrew

I

Iaan
Meaning: God is gracious
Origin: English

Isaiah
Meaning: Salvation of God
Origin: Hebrew

Itai
Meaning: God is with me
Origin: Hebrew

J

Jackie
Meaning: Likely derived from the name John meaning God is gracious
Origin: Hebrew

Jacob
Meaning: Supplanter
Origin: Hebrew

Jaden
Meaning: God has heard
Origin: Hebrew

Jaja
Meaning: Gift of God
Origin: African

Jakobe
Meaning: He who supplants
Origin: Hebrew

Jalaal
Meaning: Grandeur, glory of the faith
Origin: Arabic

James
Meaning: Supplanter/replacer
Origin: Hebrew

Janus
Meaning: Gateway
Origin: Latin

Jared
Meaning: He descends
Origin: Hebrew

Jayce
Meaning: The Lord is my salvation
Origin: Hebrew

Jazz
Meaning: Derived from Jasmine meaning gift from God
Origin: Persian

Jean-Michel
Meaning: God is gracious
Origin: Hebrew

Jedidiah
Meaning: Beloved of the Lord
Origin: Hebrew

Jeremiah
Meaning: Appointed by God
Origin: Hebrew

Jesse
Meaning: The Lord exists
Origin: Hebrew

Jibri
Meaning: Angel of Allah
Origin: African

Joachim
Meaning: Established by God
Origin: Hebrew

Joaquin
Meaning: God will judge
Origin: Spanish

Joel
Meaning: Jehovah is the Lord
Origin: Hebrew

Johann/Johan
Meaning: God is gracious
Origin: Hebrew

John
Meaning: God is gracious
Origin: Hebrew

Jojo
Meaning: God raises
Origin: Hebrew

Jonathan
Meaning: God’s gift
Origin: Hebrew

Jordan
Meaning: Flowing down
Origin: Hebrew

Josefa
Meaning: God increases
Origin: Spanish

Joseph
Meaning: God increases
Origin: Hebrew

Joshua
Meaning: The Lord is my salvation
Origin: Hebrew

Josiah
Meaning: God supports, heals
Origin: Hebrew

Judean
Meaning: Loyal to the king of Judea
Origin: Jamaican

K

Keshawn
Meaning: God is gracious
Origin: American

Keyon
Meaning: God is gracious
Origin: Irish

Kian
Meaning: God is Gracious
Origin: Irish

Kristopher
Meaning: Bearing Christ
Origin: Scandinavian

L

Lasean
Meaning: God is gracious
Origin: American

Lashawn
Meaning: God is gracious
Origin: Hebrew

Lathan
Meaning: God has given
Origin: English

Lemuel
Meaning: Devoted to God
Origin: Hebrew

M

Makai
Meaning: Who resembles God?
Origin: Hebrew

Malachi
Meaning: Messenger of God
Origin: Hebrew

Malachiah
Meaning: Messenger of God
Origin: Hebrew

Mashawn
Meaning: God is gracious
Origin: African American

Mateo
Meaning: Gift from God
Origin: Hebrew

Mathias
Meaning: Gift of God
Origin: Hebrew

Matthew
Meaning: Gift of God
Origin: Hebrew

Mawuli
Meaning: There is a God
Origin: African–Ghana

Messiah
Meaning: Anointed
Origin: Hebrew/English

Micah
Meaning: Who is like God?
Origin: Hebrew

Michael
Meaning: Who is like God?
Origin: Hebrew

Mikael
Meaning: Who is like God?
Origin: Unknown

Mikaili
Meaning: Who is like God?
Origin: African

Misha
Meaning: Who resembles God?
Origin: Hebrew

Moses
Meaning: To draw out (of water)
Origin: Hebrew

Mykel
Meaning: Who is like God?
Origin: Hebrew

N

Nate
Meaning: God has given
Origin: Hebrew

Nathan
Meaning: Gift of God
Origin: Hebrew

Nathaniel
Meaning: Gift of God
Origin: Hebrew

Nathi
Meaning: God is with us
Origin: African

Noel
Meaning: Born on Christmas
Origin: French

Nuru
Meaning: Filled with light
Origin: African-Swahili

O

Osahar
Meaning: God hears me
Origin: African

Osakwe
Meaning: The Lord agrees
Origin: African

Osayaba
Meaning: The Lord forgives
Origin: African

Osaze
Meaning: Loved by God
Origin: African-Nigeria

Ozias
Meaning: Strength from the Lord
Origin: Greek

Ozzy
Meaning: God's power
Origin: German

P

Pascal
Meaning: Easter
Origin: Latin/French

Paseka
Meaning: Easter/Born on Easter
Origin: African

Pason
Meaning: Uprising, son of God
Origin: Arabic

Paul
Meaning: Small, humble
Origin: Latin

Pelabo
Meaning: Lightning
Origin: Arabic

Pelumi
Meaning: God is with me
Origin: African–Nigeria

Peter
Meaning: Stone, rock
Origin: Greek

Philip
Meaning: Lover of horses
Origin: Greek

Psalm
Meaning: Song
Origin: Greek

Q

Qeshaun
Meaning: God is merciful
Origin: English

R

Rafael
Meaning: God has healed
Origin: Hebrew/Spanish

Raffiel
Meaning: God has healed
Origin: Unknown

Raphael
Meaning: God has healed
Origin: Hebrew

Rashon
Meaning: God is gracious
Origin: American

S

Saint
Meaning: Holy person
Origin: American

Selasi
Meaning: God hears me
Origin: African

Shawn
Meaning: God is gracious
Origin: Irish

Shawn/Sean
Meaning: God is gracious
Origin: Irish

Shia
Meaning: Praise God
Origin: Hebrew

T

Tadiwanashe
Meaning: We are loved by God
Origin: African

Teo
Meaning: God
Origin: Mexican

Theo
Meaning: God
Origin: Greek

Theodore
Meaning: Gift of God
Origin: Greek

Theophilus
Meaning: Friend of God
Origin: Latin

Tian
Meaning: Heaven
Origin: Unknown

Timeus
Meaning: To honor God
Origin: Greek

Tyrel
Meaning: God of battle
Origin: Irish

U

Uba
Meaning: Lord
Origin: African

Uriah
Meaning: God is light
Origin: Hebrew

Uzair
Meaning: Helper, strength
Origin: Arabic

Uzziah
Meaning: Jesus is my strength
Origin: Hebrew

V

Vashni
Meaning: The second
Origin: Hebrew

Vasim
Meaning: Graceful and good-looking
Origin: Arabic

W

Wali
Meaning: Lord
Origin: Arabic

Y

Yechezkel
Meaning: God strengthens
Origin: Hebrew

Yoav
Meaning: God is father
Origin: Hebrew

Yoseph
Meaning: Derived from Joseph meaning God will multiply
Origin: Hebrew

Z

Zachary

Meaning: The Lord has remembered
Origin: Hebrew

Zayne

Meaning: God is gracious
Origin: Hebrew

Zeke

Meaning: God strengthens
Origin: Hebrew

Zephan

Meaning: Hidden by God
Origin: Hebrew

Zephaniah

Meaning: God has hidden
Origin: Hebrew

GENDER-NEUTRAL NAMES A-Z BY CATEGORY

POSITIVE MEANING

"Happiness is a mood. Positivity is a mindset."

Gender Neutral ♀♂

A

Akira
Meaning: Bright, intelligent, clear
Origin: Japanese

Austin
Meaning: Great
Origin: Unknown

B

Bali
Meaning: Strength
Origin: Indonesian

Beau
Meaning: Beautiful
Origin: French

Bobby/Bobbie
Meaning: Famous, bright
Origin: German

C

Cairo
Meaning: Victorious
Origin: Arabic

D

Dayo
Meaning: Happiness has come
Origin: African

E

Emerson
Meaning: Brave, powerful
Origin: British

G

Gene
Meaning: Born lucky
Origin: Greek

Ghalen
Meaning: Calm
Origin: Greek

Gonza
Meaning: Love
Origin: Unknown

J

Jazz
Meaning: Derived from Jasmine meaning gift from God
Origin: Persian

K

Kalei
Meaning: The beloved
Origin: Hawaiian

Kamari
Meaning: Great joy
Origin: American

Katlego
Meaning: Success
Origin: African

Kay
Meaning: Pure
Origin: Unknown

Khari
Meaning: Kingly
Origin: Swahili

Kimani
Meaning: Adventurer
Origin: African

Kinta
Meaning: Laughter
Origin: Aboriginal

Kioko
Meaning: Born with happiness
Origin: Japanese

Kirabo
Meaning: Gift from God
Origin: African

Kisembo
Meaning: Gift
Origin: African–Uganda

L

Lerato
Meaning: Song of my soul, to adore a person
Origin: African

Lux
Meaning: Light
Origin: Latin

M

Magic
Meaning: Full of wonder
Origin: American

Maia
Meaning: Great
Origin: Latin

Mhina
Meaning: Delightful
Origin: African–Bakongo of Zaire

N

Neo/Neyo
Meaning: Gift
Origin: African Origin/American

Ntsako
Meaning: Joy, happiness
Origin: African–Tsonga of Central Africa

O

Orlando
Meaning: Famous throughout the land
Origin: Unknown

Q

Quinlan
Meaning: Very strong
Origin: Irish

R

Reagan
Meaning: Little king
Origin: Irish

Reese
Meaning: Enthusiastic
Origin: Welsh

Reilly
Meaning: Courageous
Origin: Irish

Royal
Meaning: The king
Origin: English

Rufaro
Meaning: Happiness
Origin: Africa–Zimbabwe

Russom
Meaning: One who is a leader
Origin: Swahili

S

Sanyu
Meaning: Happiness
Origin: African

Saphir
Meaning: Sapphire, gem
Origin: Biblical

Selam
Meaning: Peace
Origin: African

Skylar
Meaning: Scholar
Origin: Dutch

T

Tariro
Meaning: Hope
Origin: African

Tata
Meaning: Cheerful
Origin: Unknown

Tene
Meaning: One who is much loved
Origin: African

Teshi
Meaning: Cheerful
Origin: African

Tiwa
Meaning: One who owns the crown
Origin: African

Tomi
Meaning: Rich
Origin: Japanese

Tony/Toni
Meaning: Worthy of praise
Origin: Latin

Z

Zana
Meaning: Wise
Origin: Kurdish

Zen
Meaning: Meditation
Origin: Japanese

Zene
Meaning: Beautiful
Origin: African–Nigeria

Ziza
Meaning: Splendor, abundance
Origin: Biblical/Hebrew

Zohar
Meaning: Brilliance
Origin: Hebrew

SPACE & NATURE

"Shoot for the moon. Even if you miss, you'll land in the stars."

Gender Neutral ♀♂

A

Arden
Meaning: Great forest
Origin: Latin

B

Blair
Meaning: Field, plain
Origin: Scottish

Brook
Meaning: Water, stream
Origin: English

Brooklyn
Meaning: Beautiful brook
Origin: Unknown

C

Citana
Meaning: Star in the sky
Origin: Native American

D

Damani
Meaning: Tomorrow
Origin: American

Derry
Meaning: Oak grove
Origin: Irish

E

Elon

Meaning: Oak tree
Origin: Hebrew

Ennis

Meaning: Island
Origin: Irish

G

Galaxy

Meaning: Large system of stars
Origin: American

H

Hayden

Meaning: Hay valley
Origin: English

I

Ixia

Meaning: South African flower
Origin: African

J

Juno

Meaning: Youth. Also a NASA space probe orbiting Jupiter
Origin: Latin

K

Kaito

Meaning: Ocean
Origin: Unknown

L

Lake

Meaning: Body of water
Origin: British

M

Marlow

Meaning: Driftwood
Origin: British

Meadow

Meaning: Field of grass
Origin: American

N

Nash

Meaning: Dweller by the ash tree
Origin: English

North

Meaning: North
Origin: British

Nyeleti

Meaning: Star
Origin: African

O

Ocean

Meaning: Sea
Origin: Greek

Ohio

Meaning: Great river
Origin: Native American

P

Parker

Meaning: Keeper of the park
Origin: English

Phoenix

Meaning: Dark red
Origin: Greek

R

Rio

Meaning: River
Origin: Spanish

River

Meaning: Stream of water that flows to the sea
Origin: English

Rocket

Meaning: A jet propelled tube
Origin: English

Ruby

Meaning: A deep red precious stone
Origin: Latin

S

Safari

Meaning: Journey
Origin: African

Satima

Meaning: Young bull
Origin: African

Sidney

Meaning: Wide meadow
Origin: English

Soleil

Meaning: Sun
Origin: French

Star

Meaning: Luminous astronomical object
Origin: Greek

Stormy

Meaning: Impetuous nature
Origin: American

T

Timber

Meaning: Wood
Origin: English

W

Wainani

Meaning: Beautiful water
Origin: Hawaiian

Winter

Meaning: Cold Season
Origin: American

AFRICAN ORIGIN

"If we stand tall, it's because we stand on the shoulders of our ancestors." -African Proverb

Gender Neutral 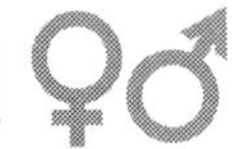

A

Africa
Meaning: From Africa
Origin: African

Akande
Meaning: First born
Origin: African–Yoruba

Anesu
Meaning: God is with us
Origin: African–Zimbabwe

Ayo
Meaning: happiness,joy
Origin: African–Nigeria

B

Banji
Meaning: Second born wwin
Origin: African

C

Chikelu
Meaning: Created by God
Origin: African

Chikere
Meaning: Created by God
Origin: African

D

Dayo
Meaning: Happiness has come
Origin: African

Deka
Meaning: Pleasing
Origin: African

Dembe
Meaning: Peace
Origin: African

Diara
Meaning: Gift
Origin: African

Dumi
Meaning: The inspirer
Origin: African

E

Ebele
Meaning: Mercy, kindness
Origin: African

Ebere
Meaning: One who shows mercy
Origin: African

Ekene
Meaning: Praise
Origin: African

Ezinwene
Meaning: Good brothers/ good sisters
Origin: African

F

Farai
Meaning: Rejoice, be happy
Origin: African

G

Gonza
Meaning: Love
Origin: African

I

Ixia
Meaning: South African flower
Origin: African

J

Jenue
Meaning: From Jenue in Nigeria
Origin: African

Jirani
Meaning: Neighbor
Origin: Swahili

Jumoke
Meaning: Everyone loves the child
Origin: African

K

Kabili
Meaning: Brave
Origin: African

Kagiso
Meaning: Peace
Origin: African

Katlego
Meaning: Success
Origin: African

Keita
Meaning: Blessing
Origin: African

Kenyatta
Meaning: Musician
Origin: African

Khari
Meaning: Kingly
Origin: Swahili

Kifimbo
Meaning: Very thin child
Origin: African

Kijana
Meaning: Youth
Origin: African

Kimani
Meaning: Adventurer
Origin: African

Kione
Meaning: Someone who comes from nowhere
Origin: African

Kirabo
Meaning: Gift from God
Origin: African

Kisembo
Meaning: Gift
Origin: African

Kitoko
Meaning: Beautiful
Origin: African

Kwayera
Meaning: Dawn
Origin: African

L

Lerato
Meaning: Song of my soul, to adore a person
Origin: African

M

Makondo
Meaning: War
Origin: African

Mashaka
Meaning: Trouble
Origin: African

Mhina
Meaning: Delightful
Origin: African

Mikaili
Meaning: Who is like God?
Origin: African

Mikenna
Meaning: Who brings joy
Origin: African

Minana
Meaning: Miracle
Origin: African–Bantu of Zimbabwe

Mufaro
Meaning: Happiness
Origin: African–Zimbabwe

N

Nalo
Meaning: Loveable
Origin: African

Naserian
Meaning: The lucky one
Origin: African

Natine
Meaning: Of the Natine tribe
Origin: African

Ndidi
Meaning: Patience
Origin: African–Nigeria

Ngoni
Meaning: Mercy
Origin: African–Zimbabwe

Ntsako
Meaning: Joy, happiness
Origin: African–Tsonga of Central Africa

Nyeleti
Meaning: Star
Origin: African

O

Ogochukwu
Meaning: The favor of God
Origin: African–Nigeria

Okal
Meaning: To cross
Origin: African

Okoth
Meaning: Born When It Was Raining
Origin: African

Olajuwon
Meaning: Wealth and honor are God's gifts
Origin: African–Nigerian

Olushola
Meaning: God has blessed or honored me
Origin: African–Nigeria

Onaedo
Meaning: Gold
Origin: African–Nigeria

Oratilwe
Meaning: Loved one
Origin: African

P

Penda
Meaning: Love
Origin: African–Swahili

R

Rafiki
Meaning: Friend
Origin: African

Rudo
Meaning: Love
Origin: African–Zimbabwe

Rufaro
Meaning: Happiness
Origin: African–Zimbabwe

Russom
Meaning: One who is a leader, a head of the charge
Origin: African–Swahili

Rutendo
Meaning: Faith
Origin: Africa–Zimbabwe

S

Safari
Meaning: Journey
Origin: African

Saidi
Meaning: Helper
Origin: African

Sandile
Meaning: You have increased our family
Origin: African

Sanyu
Meaning: Happiness
Origin: African

Sarki
Meaning: Chief
Origin: African

Satima
Meaning: Young bull
Origin: African

Selam
Meaning: Peace
Origin: African

Selasi
Meaning: God hears me
Origin: African

Sisi
Meaning: Born on Sunday
Origin: African

T

Taiwo
Meaning: First twin to taste the world
Origin: African

Tariro
Meaning: Hope
Origin: African

Tene
Meaning: One who is much loved
Origin: African

Teshi
Meaning: Cheerful
Origin: African

Tinashe
Meaning: God is with us
Origin: African

Tiwa
Meaning: One who owns the crown
Origin: African

V

Vuyo
Meaning: Happiness
Origin: African–South Africa

X

Xola
Meaning: Stay in peace
Origin: African–Xhosa of South Africa

Y

Yenge
Meaning: Work
Origin: African–Mende of Sierra Leone

Yohance
Meaning: God's gift
Origin: African–Hausa of West Africa

Z

Zaci
Meaning: God of fatherhood
Origin: African

Zaire
Meaning: The river that swallows other rivers
Origin: African

Zawadi
Meaning: Gift
Origin: African–Swahili

Zene
Meaning: Beautiful
Origin: African–Nigeria

Zo
Meaning: Spiritual Leader
Origin: African

Zoan
Meaning: Departure
Origin: African

BIBLICAL

"A good name is more to be desired than great wealth."–Proverbs 22:1

Gender Neutral ♀♂

A

Adriel

Meaning: The flock of God
Origin: Hebrew

E

Eden

Meaning: Place of pleasure
Origin: Hebrew

H

Harran

Meaning: A singing
Origin: Hebrew

I

Iram

Meaning: Shining
Origin: Arabic

Iscah

Meaning: To behold
Origin: Hebrew

Israel

Meaning: May God prevail
Origin: Hebrew

J

Jesse

Meaning: The Lord exists
Origin: Hebrew

S

Saphir
Meaning: Sapphire, gem
Origin: Biblical

Shiloh
Meaning: Tranquil
Origin: Hebrew

Z

Zenas
Meaning: Hospitable
Origin: Greek

Ziza
Meaning: Splendor, abundance
Origin: Hebrew

Zohar
Meaning: Brilliance
Origin: Hebrew

INFLUENTIAL PEOPLE

"I don't know who you will be but I know you will be my everything."

Gender Neutral ♀♂

A

Aubrey

Meaning: Ruler of The Elves, Wise
Origin: French
Influential Person: Aubrey Graham (aka Drake) – Grammy award-winning rapper, actor, and entrepreneur.

B

Bobby/Bobbie

Meaning:famous, bright
Origin: German
Influential Person:"Bobbie Brown – Grammy award-winning singer and rapper.

Bobby Marshall – First Black footballer in the NFL (along with Fritz Pollard)"

C

Charlie

Meaning: Freeman
Origin: Old German
Influential Person: Bobby Marshall – First Black footballer in the NFL (along with Fritz Pollard).

D

Doris

Meaning: Gift
Origin: Greek
Influential Person: Doris Miller – The first Black American to be awarded the Navy Cross.

J

Jack

Meaning: Likely derived from the name John meaning God is gracious
Origin: Hebrew
Influential Person: Jack Johnson – First Black boxing heavyweight champion of the world.

Jackie

Meaning: Likely derived from the name John meaning God is gracious
Origin: Hebrew
Influential Person: Jackie Robinson – First Black player in Major League Baseball, winner of the National League Most Valuable Player award and civil rights activist.

Jaden

Meaning: God has heard/ Thankful One
Origin: Hebrew
Influential Person: Jaden Smith – American rapper and actor. Son of Will Smith and Jada Pinkett-Smith.

Jesse

Meaning: The Lord exists
Origin: Hebrew
Influential Person: Jesse Owens – 4 times Olympic Gold medallist and the most successful athlete at the 1936 Berlin Olympics (held in Germany when under Hitler's rule).

Joe

Meaning: God will give
Origin: Hebrew
Influential Person: Joe Louis – Professional boxer who is widely regarded as one of the best and most influential of all time.

Jordan

Meaning: Flowing down
Origin: Hebrew
Influential Person: Jordan Peele – Actor, comedian, and filmmaker. He was the first Black director to win an Academy Award for Best Original Screenplay.

K

Kyrie

Meaning: Lord
Origin: Greek
Influential Person: Kyrie Irving – American basketballer.

M

Magic

Meaning: Full of wonder
Origin: American
Influential Person: Earvin "Magic" Johnson – American professional basketball player who is widely considered the best point guard of all time.

Morgan

Meaning: Sea
Origin: Welsh
Influential Person: Morgan Freeman – Academy Award-winning actor.

N

Neo/Neyo

Meaning: Gift
Origin: African Origin/American
Influential Person: Ne-Yo (Shaffer Smith) – Grammy Award-winning singer and songwriter.

R

Ruby

Meaning: A deep red precious stone
Origin: Latin
Influential Person: Ruby Bridges – The first Black student to attend the all-White William Frantz Elementary school at the height of desegregation.

S

Sidney

Meaning: Wide meadow
Origin: English
Influential Person: Sidney Poitier – The first Black actor to win an Academy Award.

POPULAR

"Remember that a person's name is to that person the sweetest and most important sound in any language."

Gender Neutral ♀♂

A

Africa
Meaning: From Africa
Origin: African

Akio
Meaning: Bright, clear
Origin: Japanese

Alexis
Meaning: Helper, defender
Origin: Greek

B

Bali
Meaning: Strength
Origin: Indonesia

Blair
Meaning: Field, plain
Origin: Scottish

C

Cairo
Meaning: Victorious
Origin: Arabic

Carey
Meaning: From the fort
Origin: irish

Casey
Meaning: Vigilant
Origin: Gaelic

Courtney
Meaning: From the court
Origin: English

D

Dayo
Meaning: Happiness has come
Origin: African

Delta
Meaning: Born fourth
Origin: Greek

Deon

Meaning: God
Origin: Greek

E

Elon

Meaning: Oak tree
Origin: Hebrew

G

Ghana

Meaning: A country in Africa. The word means "warrior king"
Origin: African

I

Ixia

Meaning: South African flower
Origin: African

J

Jade

Meaning: Stone of the side
Origin: Spanish

Jaden

Meaning: God has heard
Origin: Hebrew

Joe

Meaning: God will give
Origin: Hebrew

Jordan

Meaning: Flowing down
Origin: Hebrew

K

Khari

Meaning: Kingly
Origin: African–Swahili

Kyle

Meaning: Narrow
Origin: Scottish

Kyo

Meaning: Apricot
Origin: Unknown

L

Logan

Meaning: Little hollow
Origin: Scottish

M

Maia

Meaning: Great
Origin: Latin

N

Neo/Neyo

Meaning: Gift
Origin: African/American

Noel

Meaning: Born on Christmas
Origin: French

O

Ocean

Meaning: Sea
Origin: Greek

P

Phoenix
Meaning: Dark red
Origin: Greek

Psalm
Meaning: Song
Origin: Greek

R

Rayne
Meaning: Song
Origin: Scandinavian

Remi
Meaning: Oarsman
Origin: French

Riley
Meaning: Courageous
Origin: British

Rio
Meaning: River
Origin: Spanish

Ruby
Meaning: A deep red precious stone
Origin: Latin

S

Saint
Meaning: Holy person
Origin: American

Shiloh
Meaning: Tranquil
Origin: Hebrew

Stormy
Meaning: Impetuous nature
Origin: American

W

Winter

Meaning: Cold season
Origin: American

Z

Zariah

Meaning: Radiance
Origin: Arabic

Zen

Meaning: Meditation
Origin: Japanese

ARABIC

"And when the heart loves something, the eyes see it as Paradise."

Gender Neutral 

A

Aman
Meaning: Security, peace
Origin: Arabic

Amana
Meaning: Security, peace
Origin: Arabic

Amani
Meaning: Wishes
Origin: Arabic

Ara
Meaning: King, brings rain
Origin: Arabic

C

Cairo
Meaning: Victorious
Origin: Arabic

M

Manal
Meaning: Attainment
Origin: Arabic

U

Ulema
Meaning: Intelligent one
Origin: Arabic

AFRICAN AMERICAN

"Children are the reward of life."–African Proverb

Gender Neutral ♀♂

J

Jamaa

Meaning: Supplanter
Origin: Hebrew

L

Lasean

Meaning: God is gracious
Origin: American

N

Neo/Neyo

Meaning: Gift
Origin: African/American

R

Raimy

Meaning: Celebration
Origin: American

Reshay

Meaning: A gift
Origin: Jamaican

Ricki

Meaning: Brave ruler
Origin: American

T

Tinashe

Meaning: God is with us
Origin: African

MODERN

"Words have meanings. Names have power."

Gender Neutral 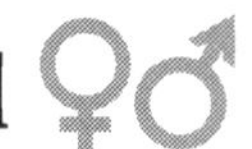

A

Ahanti

Meaning: Eternal, indestructible, warlike
Origin: Hindi

Alexis

Meaning: Helper, defender
Origin: Greek

Alyssa

Meaning: Noble
Origin: English

Aoko

Meaning: Blue child
Origin: Japanese

Ara

Meaning: King, brings rain
Origin: Arabic

Armani

Meaning: Warrior
Origin: Italian

Avery

Meaning: Ruler of the elves, wise
Origin: French

B

Bailey

Meaning: Agent of the law
Origin: Old English

Beau

Meaning: Beautiful
Origin: French

Boston

Meaning: By the woods
Origin: Unknown

Bron

Meaning: Brown, dark
Origin: French

Brooklyn

Meaning: Beautiful brook
Origin: Unknown

C

Carey
Meaning: From the fort
Origin: irish

Chase
Meaning: Huntsman
Origin: French

Chicago
Meaning: Onion
Origin: Unknown

Cosmo
Meaning: Harmony, order
Origin: Italian

D

Dallas
Meaning: The meadow dwelling
Origin: Unknown

Devon
Meaning: From Devonshire
Origin: English

Dion
Meaning: Divine
Origin: Greek

Dior
Meaning: Golden
Origin: French

Dune
Meaning: Brown skinned soldier
Origin: Scottish

E

Eden
Meaning: Place of pleasure
Origin: Hebrew

Elois
Meaning: Famous warrior
Origin: German

Elvan
Meaning: Colorful
Origin: Turkish

F

Fifi
Meaning: Jehovah increases
Origin: French

Flynn
Meaning: Son of the red-haired one
Origin: Irish

G

Gene
Meaning: Born lucky
Origin: Greek

Ghana
Meaning: A country in Africa. The word means "warrior king"
Origin: African

H

Harper
Meaning: Harp player
Origin: English

Hayden
Meaning: Hay valley
Origin: English

I

Israel
Meaning: May God prevail
Origin: Unknown

J

Jalen
Meaning: Tranquil
Origin: American

Janus
Meaning: Gateway
Origin: Latin

Jay
Meaning: Blue crested bird
Origin: Latin

Jazz
Meaning: Derived from Jasmine meaning gift from God
Origin: Persian

Jenue
Meaning: From Jenue in Nigeria
Origin: African

Jet
Meaning: Black stone
Origin: British

Jojo
Meaning: God raises
Origin: Hebrew

Judge
Meaning: Decision maker
Origin: English

Jules
Meaning: Youthful
Origin: French

K

Karma
Meaning: Fate, destiny
Origin: Sanskrit

Kaya
Meaning: Rock
Origin: Turkish

Kaylen
Meaning: Keeper of the keys
Origin: English

Kei
Meaning: Joyful
Origin: Japanese

Kendal
Meaning: Valley of the river Kent
Origin: English

Kian
Meaning: God is Gracious
Origin: Irish

Kingston
Meaning: King's settlement
Origin: British

Kione
Meaning: Someone who comes from nowhere
Origin: African

Kyrie
Meaning: Lord
Origin: Greek

L

Lamu
Meaning: Land
Origin: Unknown

Legend
Meaning: Story, myth
Origin: English

Lenka
Meaning: Torch of light
Origin: Greek

Logan
Meaning: Little hollow
Origin: Scottish

London
Meaning: From the great river
Origin: Latin

Lux
Meaning: Light
Origin: Latin

Lynx
Meaning: Brightness
Origin: Greek

M

Madison
Meaning: Gift from God
Origin: English

Magic
Meaning: Full of wonder
Origin: American

Melea
Meaning: Complete, full
Origin: Hebrew

Merritt
Meaning: Boundary gate
Origin: English

Moana
Meaning: Ocean, Sea
Origin: Hawaiian

Montell
Meaning: My ruler
Origin: French

O

Orlando

Meaning: Famous throughout the land
Origin: Unknown

P

Palmer

Meaning: Pilgrim
Origin: English

Q

Quetzal

Meaning: Large brilliant tail feather
Origin: American

Quinn

Meaning: Descendant of Conn
Origin: Irish

R

Raimy

Meaning: Celebration
Origin: American

Rain

Meaning: Rain
Origin: British

Reagan

Meaning: Little king
Origin: Irish

Reed

Meaning: Red
Origin: British

Reese

Meaning: Enthusiastic
Origin: Welsh

River

Meaning: Stream of water that flows to the sea
Origin: English

Robin
Meaning: Famous, bright
Origin: German

Rocket
Meaning: A jet propelled tube
Origin: English

Ruby
Meaning: A deep red precious stone
Origin: Latin

Ryder
Meaning: Horseman, rider
Origin: English

S

Safari
Meaning: Journey
Origin: African

Saint
Meaning: Holy person
Origin: American

Santana
Meaning: Follower of St. Ana
Origin: Spanish

Sisi
Meaning: Born on Sunday
Origin: African

Sloan
Meaning: Warrior
Origin: Scottish

Stacy
Meaning: Resurrection
Origin: English

Storm
Meaning: Tempest
Origin: British

T

Taiwo
Meaning: First twin to taste the world
Origin: African

Tokyo
Meaning: Eastern capital
Origin: Unknown

V

Vale
Meaning: Lives in the valley
Origin: Latin

Vanya
Meaning: God is gracious
Origin: Slavic

Veda
Meaning: Knowledge or wisdom
Origin: Sanskrit

X

Xochitl
Meaning: Flower
Origin: Aztec

Y

Yonah
Meaning: Dove
Origin: Unknown

CLASSIC

"A good name will shine forever."

Gender Neutral ♀♂

A

Andy

Meaning: Manly
Origin: Greek

C

Courtney

Meaning: From the court
Origin: English

J

Jackie

Meaning: Likely derived from the name John meaning God is gracious
Origin: Hebrew

Joe

Meaning: God will give
Origin: Hebrew

P

Pearl

Meaning: Pearl
Origin: Unknown

R

Ryan

Meaning: Little king
Origin: Irish

RELIGIOUS

"Babies are a bit of stardust blown from the hands of God."

Gender Neutral ♀♂

A

Arie

Meaning: Lion of God
Origin: Hebrew

C

Cyrille

Meaning: Lord
Origin: Unknown

D

Damani

Meaning: Tomorrow
Origin: American

Deon

Meaning: God
Origin: Greek

Dominique

Meaning: Of the Lord
Origin: Latin

H

Haskell

Meaning: God's helmet
Origin: Norse

J

Jackie
Meaning: Likely derived from the name John meaning God is gracious
Origin: Hebrew

Jaden
Meaning: God has heard
Origin: Hebrew

Janus
Meaning: Gateway
Origin: Latin

Jazz
Meaning: Derived from Jasmine meaning gift from God
Origin: Persian

Jesse
Meaning: The Lord exists
Origin: Hebrew

Jojo
Meaning: God raises
Origin: Hebrew

Jordan
Meaning: Flowing down
Origin: Hebrew

K

Kian
Meaning: God is Gracious
Origin: Irish

L

Lasean
Meaning: God is gracious
Origin: American

M

Mikaili
Meaning: Who is like God?
Origin: African

Misha
Meaning: Who resembles God?
Origin: Hebrew

N

Noel
Meaning: Born on Christmas
Origin: French

Nuru
Meaning: Filled with light
Origin: Swahili

P

Pascal
Meaning: Easter
Origin: Latin/French

Psalm
Meaning: Song
Origin: Greek

S

Saint
Meaning: Holy person
Origin: American

Selasi
Meaning: God hears me
Origin: African

NOTES

When you find a name you like, shortlist here. Make a note of the name, page number, meaning & and anything else that makes the name a contender. This way you can simply compare your options to help you make a final decision more easily.

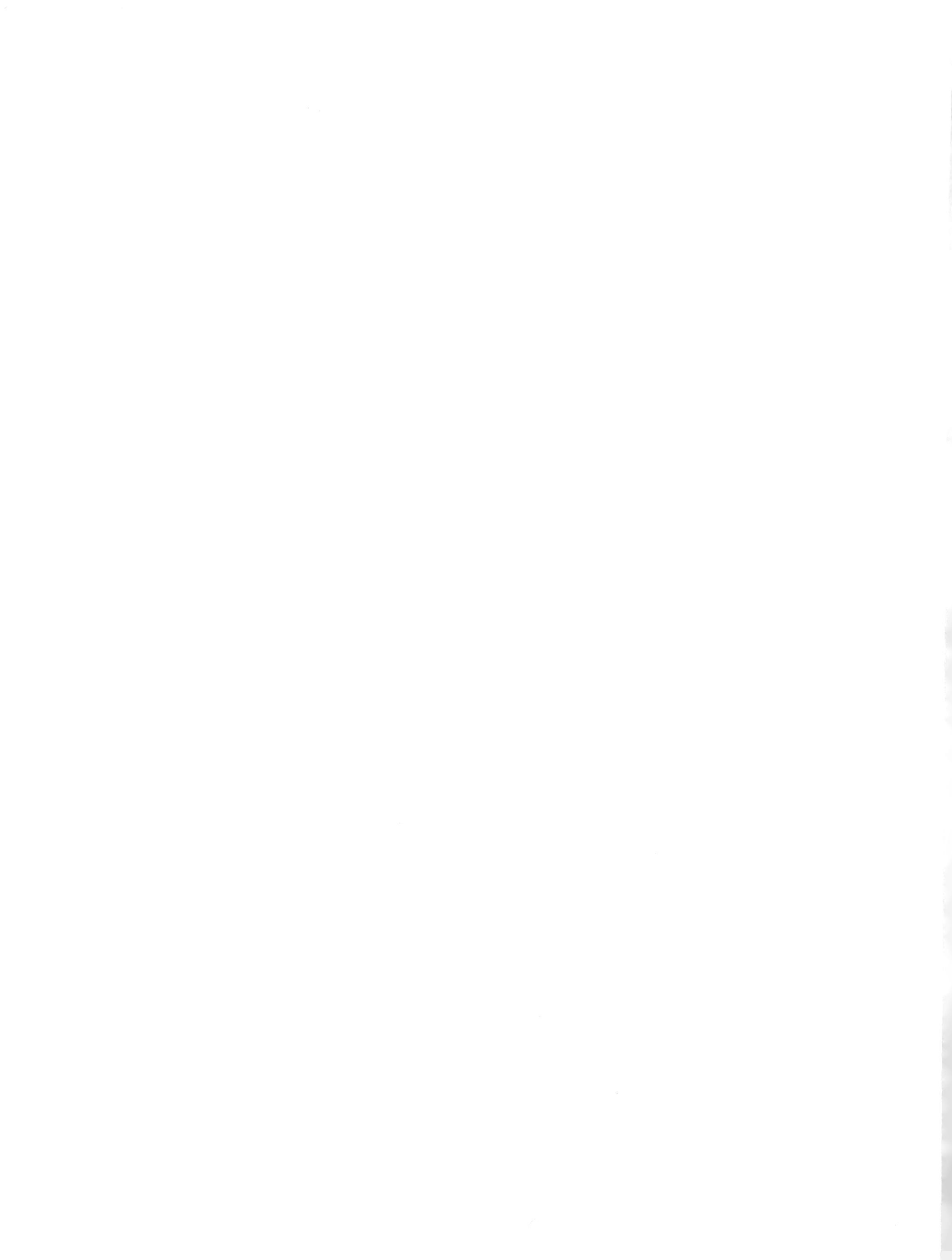

Made in the USA
Columbia, SC
16 November 2022